MW01028550

18 Weeks

TO A

HEALTHIER, HAPPIER, More Purposeful Life

LACY NGO

ISBN: 978-1-957723-58-7 (hard cover)
      978-1-957723-59-4 (soft cover)

Edited by: Melissa Long

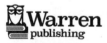

Published by WARREN Publishing
Charlotte, NC
www.warrenpublishing.net
Printed in the United States

For my mom and dad, my husband, Chad,
and my children, Hilt and Neeshie

ACKNOWLEDGMENTS

I am forever grateful to my husband for supporting me and rooting for me as I spent years researching and writing. I'd also like to thank my parents for being my biggest cheerleaders and my children for teaching me to enjoy the simple things in life. I also want to say a special thank you to my book club girls. At each book club gathering, I discovered something new about life, God's love, and myself. Finally, I would like to thank Warren Publishing and my publishing team, Mindy, Amy, Melissa, Monika, and Audrey, for elevating my book to a place I never thought it could reach.

ACKNOWLEDGMENTS

TABLE OF CONTENTS

ABOUT THE AUTHOR

Lacy Ngo is a registered dietitian with a *Master's in Human Nutrition*. She is also one of the top experts in faith-based mindfulness and nutrition. Ngo is the owner of Mindfulness in Faith and Food, LLC, a faith-based nutrition website that focuses on mindful eating and mindful living. Whether it's through her blog or her books, Ngo's mission is to make healthy eating easier and more convenient for busy families living in a chaotic world. For more information, please visit her website: www.mindfulnessinfaithandfood.com.

DISCLAIMER

This book does not replace medical advice. This book contains general nutrition information from a registered dietitian. However, nutritional needs vary among individuals based on labs, medical conditions, genetics, etc. Please discuss any medical conditions one-on-one with a doctor or dietitian. A dietitian can help you personalize a diet for any specific conditions. For example, if you have diabetes, a dietitian can tailor diet recommendations specifically to your condition. This book is not liable or responsible if someone takes advice from this book and has any problems.

PART 1
THE IMPACT (THE *WHY*)

*A*fter experiencing a different way of living, I wanted to shout it out to everyone: *this new approach has changed me!* What if these simple, daily, faith-based, mindful techniques could help others? Help *you*? With these questions in mind, I decided I wanted to share my techniques with you in this easy-to-follow, eighteen-week plan. I pray that this program helps you experience life and wellness in a whole new way. Each week, I encourage you to read a chapter and try to incorporate the weekly challenge into your daily life. Each challenge is meant to improve your health and add joy and purpose to your everyday life.

LESSON 1

Mindful Living and Eating: An Introduction

The Weight-Obsessing Begins

When I was in middle school, I was teased for being on the heavier side. "Here comes the two-ton whale" is one comment that still frequently flashes through my mind. This comment was what pushed me into my weight obsession. Fueled by embarrassment, I lost weight, but in the process, I became weight-obsessed. I stopped eating breakfast and lunch, but I still ate dinner since I ate it with my family. Obviously, they never knew I wasn't eating any other meal, and since I was only eating dinner with them, they had no reason to know. I would run or do a workout video every day when I got home from school. I had headaches most of the day and was always hungry, but I was losing weight, so I pushed through.

I was proud of my weight loss and maintained my "ideal" body weight all through middle school, high school, and college. I felt good in my clothes. No one made fun of me, and, suddenly, the boys who had teased me were now flirting with me. The sad truth is I was treated better by others at school after I lost weight. Life seemed better when I was smaller, and I wanted to help others achieve their weight-loss goals as well. In fact, I decided to get my degree in human nutrition so I could help others lose weight too. As I worked to get my master's in human nutrition, I learned food could do amazing things for us—later, I will share these amazing things, and I hope you are as amazed as I am—and health was not all about weight loss. Yet I was still weight-obsessed. I didn't want life to go back to the way it was when I was heavier. I didn't want to be treated the way I was treated when I was heavier. So even after everything I had learned, I continued to focus on weight. Once I got my degree, I finally understood how impactful nutrients from God's earth are to our health, *and* I became familiar with the best evidence-based weight loss practices. As you can guess, I focused on the latter.

Mindful Eating Changed My Focus

Early in my career as a dietitian, I started reading about an up-and-coming technique in our field called "mindful eating." This technique intrigued me. *You mean, I don't have to follow all these food rules or keep up the willpower?* This way of eating sounded so freeing to me! Dietitians must take continuing education units throughout their careers to keep their dietetics license. So for one of my continuing education courses, I decided to take a Mindful Eating for Dietitians course. During this course, we were asked to go through a mindful-eating exercise. I never knew I could enjoy food so much or could feel so satisfied after eating.

What's Not to Love?

I loved everything about mindful eating! No willpower was needed, and no food was off limits. I could just enjoy my food. Yet mindful eating was about much more than just slowly eating whatever you want. Mindful eating was about pausing before each bite *and* listening to your body before making food choices. Mindful eating was about learning what the science says about food and noticing how your body reacts when you apply that science to your eating. Mindful-eating was about focusing on the other things food could do for you other than just helping with weight control—although if weight loss is beneficial, mindful eating does help with weight loss as well. What's not to love?

If all of this seems confusing to you, don't worry. Later in this book, you will find a step-by-step guide explaining what this pause looks like and how we can listen to our bodies and apply the science when eating and making food choices.

Adding Faith to Mindful Eating

One of the biggest components of mindful eating is the pause, and since I am a person of faith, I naturally incorporated my faith into my mindful-eating pause. Pausing sets the stage for the whole eating experience. Pausing gets your mind ready to mindfully eat. When I paused and looked at my food, I automatically began to thank God for the miracle of food. During the pause, I began to realize how miraculous food really was. Our bodies can't thrive on their own; they need certain things found in food to flourish. And, miraculously, we can get these "things"—quercetin, anthocyanin antioxidants, omega-3s, vitamin c, zinc, fiber, L-theanine and other amino acids, and energy that help our moods, brains, and energy levels—from the foods we eat!

Faith-Based Mindful Eating Changed My Health

I never could have imagined how much faith-based mindfulness and nutrition would impact my health, but, wow, did it ever! My mood and stress levels improved within weeks, and my asthma and seasonal allergies became almost nonexistent. Before transforming my approach to food, I would get a terrible, debilitating cough and mucus drainage for weeks every fall and spring like clockwork.

After incorporating this way of eating and living, I didn't get the cough or mucus drainage for the first time in, well, *ever*! Did you know that research shows nutrition can even impact seasonal allergies? Don't worry, we'll talk more about everything food can do for us later.

Anyway, that wasn't the only change. Ironically, I even lost weight—about fifty pounds—even though I was no longer focusing on weight. My forty-year-old body can now do more than it could do in my twenties. I can run and play with my children without getting tired. I can walk at an amusement park all day long and still have the energy to go for a run afterward if I want to. I can paddleboard for miles, speed through the monkey bars, and carry loads of groceries into my house at one time. I can hold up cabinets as my husband, Chad, installs them or carry my seven-year-old on a walking trail for a mile when she gets tired. I no longer have hip pain when I run, and even my acne went away. I had acne since middle school and saw a dermatologist regularly. I continued to have acne as an adult ... until I changed my eating. Now my acne has improved by leaps and bounds.

Since I am the main chef at home, I made changes to our meals and saw a positive impact in my family as well. My children's behavior improved, and my son's asthma became almost untraceable. Moreover, my son used to have a short temper. He would get frustrated and mad quickly. He would yell and slam doors when he was angry—I yelled more often, too, before changing my way of eating and living. I haven't seen him lose his temper in that way since we started eating and living more mindfully. He even noticed an increase in his speed and endurance when he played soccer.

Throughout all these changes, I was connecting more with God while I ate my food. I focused on God and His gift of food throughout the meal. When I focus on God more, I notice His presence and am more appreciative of His blessing. I also "hear" Him whisper more when I am taking the time to notice.

Mindful Eating Evolved to Mindful Living

Something even more beautiful happened as well. I noticed how much pausing before eating helped me, and I started to think: *What if I incorporated aspects of faith-based mindful eating into my whole life?*

So I decided to start pausing and praying before entering any new environment. I paused and prayed before going into my children's school or the grocery store or the bank. Let's use the bank as an example. When I entered the bank, I focused on my surroundings and the people in the bank. As I prayed, I remembered that these people in *this* bank are the people God put into my life in this very moment, and I wanted to be present with them and love them. When I took the time to notice and love others, I really *saw* them and had compassion and patience for my brothers and sisters. The bottom line: I was kinder to others when I remembered how precious every human being I met was. And pausing and praying before entering a new environment gave me time to listen for God's guidance, His whisper. The Bible encourages us to continuously pray, and I felt like pausing and praying before entering a new place was a way for me to do just that.

Mindful Living Led to More Goosebump Moments

The story doesn't end there.

When I added this mindful prayer before entering any new place to my routine, something surprisingly wonderful happened. I started noticing God more and experiencing amazing goosebump moments all over the place. All because I was taking the time to notice God and His presence! Because I took the time to notice, I now have a multitude of these "goosebump stories" to share, and every time I share one of them, people react in awe, often showing me the chills on their arms. Keep reading because I have included many of these stories in this study. They can be found in part 3.

Discussion Questions

1. Do you have any "goosebump stories" in which you were in awe of God's presence? Would you like to share your story or how you felt after having the experience?
2. 1 Thessalonians 5:16–18 (English Standard Version) says, "Rejoice always, pray without ceasing, give thanks in all circumstances; for this is the will of God in Christ Jesus for you." What does this Bible verse mean to you? How do you think you can honor this verse in your own life?
3. Do you think praying before entering any new place would help you notice God's presence more often?

Weekly Challenge

1. Pray before entering any new environment this week. We will discuss your experiences next week.

LESSON 2
Faith-Based Mindful Eating

Our bodies are amazing. God gave us everything we need to flourish, and He gave us bodies that can tell us what we need. We should listen, for these signals are a beautiful gift from God. When we feel cold, we reach for the nearby blanket; when we feel hot, we look for shade or air conditioning; and when we feel dirty, we crave a shower or bath. When we need to go to the bathroom, we don't tell ourselves to wait a few more hours–that sounds painful—we just go. And when we feel hungry, it is our bodies' way of saying, "It's time to eat."

In the nutrition world, this is called "intuitive eating." With intuitive eating, your body tells you when it is time to eat, and when you listen to this whisper, you usually end up the size you should be for optimal health. Please keep in mind that this size is different for everyone. Mindful eating and intuitive eating help *your* body fall into the size *your* body wants to be for optimal health.

Mindful Eating Changed Everything for Me
Faith-based mindful eating changed *everything* for me. Mindful eating gave me so much hope. Hope I could live life more slowly.

Hope I could fully enjoy my food and my life. Hope I could feel God's presence everywhere and in every situation. Hope I now had a strategy that would help me remember God and others more often. I now had a plan that would help me make more loving choices.

Mindfulness Was Key

For the first time, I did not need willpower to deny my cravings, push through hunger, or eat something I didn't really want. I didn't deprive myself and didn't even feel the need to have cheat days. I discovered that, for me, the most important component of mindful eating was the *pause* before and during my meals. That pause, or lack of the pause, was the determining factor in whether I would mindfully eat or not.

Why Is the Pause So Crucial?

When I pause, I remind myself to take my time, notice my food, and recognize if I am eating an amount of food that makes me feel satisfied but not overly full. I remind myself to take the time to pay attention to my food instead of overconsuming without even noticing I am eating. Most importantly, during this pause, I thank God for the food.

When I pause, I remind myself to eat God's gift of food for enjoyment *and* nourishment. When I stop to thank God for the nourishing food, I find myself *wanting* food from God's earth more than an ultra-processed snack. I find it helpful to put my fork down in between bites and completely focus on the joy of eating *that* bite. When you do this, every bite becomes an experience, and when you focus on each bite, you give your brain time to recognize that you are eating. When your brain has time to process, it has time to signal when your body is feeling full and satisfied. Eating becomes a beautiful time to relax and decompress.

Does Mindful Eating Mean You Can
Now Eat Whatever You Want?

Kind of. Life is all about balance. The correct answer to anything
in life sits somewhere in the middle. Let me explain:

- We should show kindness to those who hurt us, but we
  should also stand up when someone is being mistreated.
- When put in a parental or leadership role, we must walk
  the line between being too strict and being too lenient.
- We want to be hardworking, but too much work can
  sometimes be harmful to our bodies.
- We should strive to improve and grow, but we should also
  be proud of where we are and who we are at that moment.

Honestly, any scenario in life is about learning to balance in the
middle. Life is a balancing act. We will sway too far one way or
another from time to time, but the middle is the sweet spot. When
I was weight obsessing, I had significantly veered away from that
sweet spot. But just like everything else, we can also lean too far
the other way as well.

Does Mindfulness Let Us Eat Whatever We Want?

When we listen to our bodies and learn what the science says
about how certain foods can benefit our bodies, we often find that
"what we want" changes. Mindfulness is not only about mindfully
enjoying every bite of your food but also about being mindful of
our choices. Perhaps my body wants a less-nutrient dense food
because it brings back beautiful memories, but I also know that if I
eat that food every day, my body, mind, and mood will be affected.

So I mindfully choose to eat less nutrient-dense foods on occasion,
but on most days, I mindfully choose to eat delicious nutrient-
dense foods that are going to promote a positive mood, support my
immune system, promote cognitive function, and reduce the risk of
many diseases and conditions. For me, it wasn't until I focused on
enjoying my food through faith-based mindfulness *and* focused on

how food benefited my mind, mood, energy, and health instead of how food affected "the way I looked" that I finally stopped weight obsessing. Ironically, I have never felt healthier or happier in my own body.

What If I Still *Want* to Lose Weight?

In society, we have learned so much about the negative impact weight-obsessing and diet culture has on us. In fact, I think we are sometimes so scared about falling back into that weight-obsessed trap that we have made others feel guilty, like they are somehow wrong for still expressing a desire to lose weight. Yet people have experienced many health benefits after losing weight, such as less joint pain or improved energy. As shown in case studies and research, many have found relief and have seen significant improvements in their medical conditions after losing weight.[1] I have seen this in my clients and myself as well. So I think it's okay if you have a desire to lose weight when your desire comes from wanting to improve your health.

With that being said, I would like to encourage you to focus on what other positive impacts food can have on you other than just providing a way to lose weight. "Health" comes in many different shapes. Even if everyone ate exactly the same, we still would all be different sizes. You may be surprised to find that you feel fantastic even if you don't look like what magazines tell you to look like. And once you start mindful eating and focusing on what foods can do for your health, you may, ironically, lose weight in the process.

So like everything in life, we must try to find a good balance when it comes to "eating whatever we want" and "making healthy choices." Faith-based mindfulness as well as learning about the amazing benefits of foods helps us do just that. In fact, you may find that "eating whatever you want" and "making healthy choices" are often one in the same because, as you will see later, your desires change when you mindfully eat and mindfully choose your food based on science and cravings.

There are reasons you may desire weight loss, and fortunately mindful eating can help with weight loss while also helping you stop that food obsessing often associated with dieting. Mindful eating helps you feel full and notice your hunger/satiety cues. Moreover, the desire to binge decreases because you are actually enjoying your food *all the time*.

What Are the Benefits to Mindful Eating?

With mindful *breathing*, we are pausing and centering our minds on one thing: breathing. When we are mindfully *eating*, we are centering our brain on eating. With faith-based mindful eating, we are resting our brains by focusing on God and the food He provides.

There are benefits to resting our brain through mindful eating.[2] Did you know that stress feeds harmful bacteria in our guts? Stress alone can cause inflammation, decrease immune function, cause weight gain, and increase your risk for many chronic conditions.[3] Mindful eating can help relieve stress, promote better cognitive function, help with weight and portion control, and even improve gut health.

Mindful eating relieves stress. Mindful eating is a stress reliever.[4] Making time for mediation or quiet time can help reduce stress, but when you are super busy, finding time for such things can be hard. You have to eat anyway, so eating is a time naturally built into your day you can use to de-stress, and you can do this by mindful eating. Mindfulness is about slowing down and calming your brain. When you meditate, you center your thoughts. When you mindfully eat, you center your thoughts on eating. You try to focus on eating and nothing else; you eat slowly and taste your food. In other words, mindful eating is a time to de-stress in a busy world.

Did you know that stress feeds harmful bacteria in our gut? Stress alone can cause inflammation, decrease immune function, cause weight gain, and increase your risk for many chronic conditions.

Mindful eating promotes gut health. Mindful eating can aid in digestion.[5] How? Although most digestive enzymes are released in the stomach, digestion actually starts in the mouth. One enzyme called salivary amylase is released in the mouth. This enzyme starts breaking down carbohydrates. In fact, if you let a piece of bread sit in your mouth for a moment, you may notice a sweeter taste. That taste occurs because the more complex carbohydrate is breaking down into a simpler sugar. Chewing thoroughly helps with digestion because digestion starts in the mouth! Plus, chewing thoroughly gives the enzymes in your stomach more surface area to do their work, which again promotes healthy digestion and absorption. Anything that promotes a healthy gut sounds great to me!

Mindful eating may reduce the risk of chronic disease. Because mindful eating helps relieve stress and promotes gut health, mindful eating may reduce the risk of chronic diseases and conditions. Stress increases the risk of many chronic diseases, and poor gut health is related to inflammation and reduced immune function. Gut health, inflammation, and immunity are all linked to many conditions including IBS, Crohn's, autoimmune diseases, Alzheimer's, heart disease, stroke, brain function and focus, mood, and even depression and anxiety—to name a few.[6]

Mindful eating helps with weight loss and portion control. Although I encourage you to focus on the other benefits of mindful eating, I recognize that weight loss can be another benefit. When I mindfully focus on God's presence while eating, I do much less overeating. In fact, mindful eating has helped with portion control more than anything else I have ever tried because when you slow down and enjoy your food, you are satisfied by the amount of food your body wants and needs, which is often less than many of us are consistently eating. Seriously, I will ask you to try it soon, and when you do, you will be amazed at how full you will feel after eating a balanced plate.

Let me give you an example. Let's say you are eating dinner with a six-foot-three football player. He needs more food and devours two plates of spaghetti and three pieces of garlic bread in forty-five minutes. You eat one plate of spaghetti and half a piece of garlic bread, but it also takes you forty-five minutes. You both were able to enjoy eating for forty-five minutes, yet you are stuffed on less food than the football player. That flavorful spaghetti was in both of your mouths for the same amount of time. Would you feel like you even ate less food than the football player? Remember, I have lost fifty pounds through faith-based mindful eating.

As for focusing on God's presence while eating, doing so really helps me appreciate what these foods can do and remember that eating can be an act of worship. I will go into more detail on this practice later.

Discussion Questions

1. How do you think faith-based mindful eating would be helpful in your life?

2. 1 Corinthians 10:31 (ESV) says, "So, whether you eat or drink or whatever you do, do it all for the glory of God." How might this Bible verse relate to faith-based mindful eating?

Weekly Challenge

For this week, try adding a mindful prayer before all your meals. Focus on the gift of food in front of you and think about the nourishment in the food. Thank God for all the nourishment the food provides.

Discuss Last Week's Challenge

Last week, you were challenged to pray before entering any new environment. What are some observations you had during this experience?

LESSON 3
Faith-Based Mindful Living

The pause before and throughout the meal was crucial for my nutritional health, but I also began to notice how crucial the pause was in every aspect of my life.

As mentioned in Lesson 1, I started noticing how impactful pausing and praying before entering any new environment was in my life, whether the new environment was a park, a friend's home, or the grocery store. I also noticed the importance of pausing and praying in other times as well, like when I felt angry and almost said something mean or spoke harshly to my children. I noticed the importance of not only pausing and praying before meals and snacks, but also before I went to bed and got up in the morning. Remember, the Bible talks about praying continuously. In a way, the pause in life helps me pray more continuously because when I pause and pray before every meal, every change in environment, every time I get in the car, every conversation, or every time I type on social media, then I am praying more continuously throughout the day.

When I forget to do this, I notice the difference in *my* actions and strength to endure life. On the days when I do a better job of pausing, I notice God's presence and guidance more. When I pause more, I feel like I am truly letting God lead me, and I am reminded that no matter what happens, God is right there. I can feel God's presence with me everywhere, and I feel I have the strength to focus on God's will instead of my emotions. We don't have to rush into every situation, and we don't have to rush to speak. We can, and should, *pause* and take our time in life.

Pausing and praying had another effect as well. When I take the time to pause and be present, I am no longer too busy to *notice* God at work in my life. Consequently, I get to experience, or at least notice, many more "goosebump moments" in life—see Part 3 for some of my "goosebump" experiences.

Discussion Questions

1. What are times in your daily life when you could pause and pray?
2. How do you think pausing and praying throughout the day could benefit your life?
3. How do you think pausing and praying might help you manifest love, joy, peace, patience, kindness, goodness, faithfulness, gentleness, and self-control in your daily encounters? see Galatians 5:22–23 (ESV)

Weekly Challenge

This week's challenge is to do a mini pause and prayer before saying something in person, on the phone, in a text, in an email, or on social media.

Discussion of Last Week's Challenge

Last week, you were challenged to add a mindful prayer before all your meals. What are your observations from this challenge? In what ways, if any, was this exercise helpful to you?

LESSON 4
The Miracle of Food

Pretend you're a cartoon character in a children's show. You are walking down an alley when you notice a beautiful, sparkling door. Of course, you are going to open that door. Your breath is taken away by what you see. It's a beautiful garden filled with flowers, trees, and all kinds of natural-growing foods. A little bunny greets you as you enter. She tells you that miraculous things grow from the ground and the trees. She also tells you that the plants in this garden improve your mood, help you stay focused and alert, give you energy, and prevent disease. There are even plants that help with sleep and relaxation.

You are shocked. "Wow, I wish the food back home could do all that!"

The creature gives you a puzzled look and says, "But this is just an ordinary garden, and this stuff is in your world too."

When we really take the time to stop and think about food, we truly begin to notice just how miraculous food is. I mean, isn't it *amazing* that food resolved my severe seasonal allergy attacks and significantly improved my mood? We can get these foods that help our mood, brain, and energy levels straight out of the ground or from a tree.

Talk about a miracle! God created this earth and these foods so we could not only survive but also thrive!

Does Nutrition *Really* Have That Big of an Impact?

Before moving on, the dietitian in me must share a little research with you to drive my point home. Based on all the articles, reviews, meta-analyses, and books written by dietitians I have found and researched, the nutrients and foods discussed in this next chapter are incredibly impactful when it comes to our health. (See bibliography and additional sources for list of all my research.)

The MIND, Mediterranean, and Blue Zone diets as well as gut-healthy foods all contain these nutrients. All these diets have been shown to reduce the risk of a multitude of diseases and conditions. Moreover, the studies that were done on each individual nutrient on the list in Appendix A show the same benefits.

The Benefits of the Mediterranean and MIND Diet Based on Research

The Mediterranean and MIND diets are similar in many ways. They both encourage eating diets high in whole foods, like fruits, vegetables, whole grains, nuts, and seeds. The MIND diet emphasizes high intakes of berries since berries have been shown to protect our minds.

Dietitian and MIND diet expert Maggie Moon talks about both the Mediterranean and MIND diet in her book, *The MIND Diet*.[7] She describes how studies have shown that Mediterranean-style eating patterns are linked with a lower risk of neurodegenerative diseases like Parkinson's—and the MIND diet seems to protect against cognitive decline in aging overall. Moon writes, "The two key MIND diet studies show how the diet keeps the aging brain seven and a half years younger and reduces the risk of developing Alzheimer's disease by 53 percent."[8]

Evidence also suggests that the Mediterranean diet may be beneficial for many, *many* other conditions, like mood disorders, ADHD, cancer, asthma, and even seasonal allergies.[9] One study looked at one hundred twenty children and adolescents and found an increased prevalence of ADHD in children and adolescents who consumed a large amount of fast food, sugar, sugar-sweetened beverages, and a low amount of Mediterranean-style diet foods.[10] Yet another study found higher rates of ADHD in children who ate a diet high in processed foods, salt, and sugar and low in omega-3, fiber, and folate. Lower rates of ADHD were seen in children who had diets rich in Mediterranean-style foods, like fish, fruits, vegetables, legumes, and whole grains.[11] Studies have found that the consumption of a combination of fatty acids, omega-3s, probiotics, amino acids, vitamins, and minerals—especially magnesium, zinc, and iron—appears to improve metabolic stress markers in individuals with ADHD. Moreover, these individuals reported a reduction in emotional problems.[12]

The Mediterranean diet may decrease the frequency and severity of asthma symptoms and allergic respiratory disease.[13] Research has shown that diets low in fiber and antioxidants are associated with an increase in asthma severity.[14] The Mediterranean diet is high in fiber and antioxidants. According to research, antioxidants, like the ones often eaten in the Mediterranean diet, may also reduce the risk of developing asthma in the first place.[15]

And finally, according to a review of several studies, fiber, antioxidants, vegetables, fruits, nuts, seeds, legumes, and green tea, which are foods prevalent in the Mediterranean diet, have been shown to reduce the risk of cancer and decrease tumor cell growth.[16]

Blue Zone Foods

Researching the Blue Zone diets also provided clues to what foods I should be eating. If I want to build a business, I look to the business people who are making a profit and try to follow their lead. We use the term "benchmark" to refer to something that serves as a standard best practice. Perhaps we should do this with nutrition as well. Are there areas where people seem to be getting this "living a healthy life" thing right? Maybe we should see what they are doing and try to incorporate some of their practices into our lives.

Turns out, we already have our "healthy living" benchmark. We call these areas the Blue Zones. They refer to areas in the world where people are living long, high-quality lives. The people living in one of these five Blue Zones have lower rates of chronic disease and a higher satisfaction with their quality of life and well-being. The following are the five regions where you can find the world's longest-living people who are living without significant memory or physical problems: Loma Linda, California; Ikaria, Greece; Okinawa, Japan; Nicoya, Costa Rica; and Sardinia, Italy.[17]

So, what are these Blue Zone guys and gals doing that the rest of us aren't? Honestly, they all share several common characteristics. For one thing, their diets are 90–100 percent plant-based and consist mostly of beans, legumes, fruits, vegetables, whole grains, and nuts. They also eat small amounts of fish, lean meats, and eggs.[18] Also, the most common oil used in the Blue Zones is olive oil. They eat foods that contain natural sugar, but they rarely eat foods that contain added sugar or are heavily processed. Fermented vegetables are common in the Blue Zone areas as well and are a good source of gut health probiotics. Blue Zone folks also mainly drink water, but they also drink coffee, tea, and small amounts of red wine. Tea and red wine are packed with antioxidants, which have anti-inflammatory properties and may reduce the risk of a multitude of conditions, like heart disease, cancer, mood disorders, and Alzheimer's disease.[19]

Interestingly, along with following similar diet patterns, the people in these Blue Zones also tend to naturally practice mindful eating and are in tune with their hunger as well. Perhaps they're really onto something!

Gut Health

Our bodies naturally contain a mixture of living bacteria. Some bacteria can actually improve our health. Other bacteria ("bad" bacteria) can have a negative impact on our health. We can do things to help the "good" bacteria grow and thrive. We can also do things to decrease the bad bacteria in our bodies. Bad bacteria and good bacteria compete to occupy our bodies. So the more we nurture the good bacteria, the less bad bacteria can grow, and vice versa. A healthy gut has more "good" bacteria than "bad" bacteria and is also digesting and absorbing properly. Inversely, a leaky gut is not absorbing properly. With a leaky gut, undigested foods and bacteria leak from your intestines into your bloodstream.

In her book *Health Takes Guts,* dietitian Dianne Rishikof writes, "The influence that gut microbes have [on a person's overall health] cannot be overstated. They are the root cause and solutions to most health troubles."[20] Wow—this is a bold statement, and I understand why she makes it. I haven't decided if I'm ready to say that gut health is the "root cause" of most health conditions, but there's no question about the fact that multitudes of studies show what a huge role gut health plays in a vast number of conditions, including an array of autoimmune diseases, mood and behavioral disorders, and chronic conditions. Gut health also plays a role in weight, allergies, joint pain, and inflammation.[21]

The Research

To make sure we understand the impact of food, let's look at some of the fascinating stats I have collected over the years as a registered dietitian:

- Diet can be linked to 30 to 35 percent of cancer cases.[22]
- In one study, researchers showed that supplementation of vitamin D was associated with a 40 percent reduction in the risk of developing multiple sclerosis.[23]

- According to Marilyn Haugen and dietitian Doug Cook in *175 Best Super Food Blends Recipes*, "A diet rich in fruits, vegetables, nuts, seeds, legumes, whole grains, fish, antioxidants, and healthy herbs and spices can reduce the risk of type 2 diabetes by 90 percent and Alzheimer's by 40 percent."[24]
- In one study, elementary children who ate whole grains for breakfast versus children who only drank fruit juice scored better on standardized reading comprehension, fluency, and mathematics tests.[25]
- In another study, when children were given an antioxidant-rich fruit smoothie, they immediately reported improved moods.[26]
- Vitamin D deficiency is associated with an 8–14 percent increased risk of depression. The study also reported a higher prevalence of vitamin D deficiency among those who have attempted suicide.[27]
- Theanine and EGCG, found in green tea, may have anti-anxiety effects similar to anti-anxiety medications and may help relax the brain without making you feel drowsy.[28]
- In one study, people who drank four or more cups of green tea a day were 51 percent less likely to get depression compared to those who drank one or less per day.[29]
- Deficiencies and food intolerances can cause severe depression and even psychosis for some. In fact, in case studies, researchers found that if the patient was deficient in a nutrient, that patient's severe depression and psychosis went into complete remission after either adding supplements or omitting their food intolerances from their diets due to the patient having a food intolerance.[30]
- When older adults ate one cup of blueberries for ninety days, their memory and ability to accurately switch tasks improved compared to the placebo.[31]

- Healthy older women who consumed a combination of lutein and DHA everyday had improved verbal fluency, memory scores, and increased rates of learning after four months. Lutein is found in dark, leafy greens, and DHA is found in salmon, tuna, and other fatty fish.[32]
- Apples and citrus fruits have been shown to have a positive effect on people with asthma.[33]
- The Mediterranean diet may reduce the risk of breast cancer, colorectal cancer, and prostate cancer by approximately 60–70 percent and lung cancer by 40–50 percent.[34]
- In mice and in vitro studies, the antioxidant sulforaphane, found in broccoli and broccoli sprouts, may reduce the risk of some cancers and even the size and number of cancer cells by 50–75 percent.[35]
- In a double-blinded randomized study, prisoners who took vitamin and mineral supplements committed 26.3 percent fewer offenses compared to the prisoners who took a placebo.[36]
- In one study, a single-cup increase in vegetables—excluding nightshade vegetables, potatoes, and legumes—decreases the rate of having a multiple sclerosis relapse by 50 percent.[37]
- Studies have shown antioxidants, like flavonoids and catechins, may reduce the number of sick days by about 30–40 percent.[38]
- Adequate zinc intakes may shorten the duration of a cold by 33–44 percent.[39]

You can find more information about this data and related research articles on my website, www.mindfulnessinfaithandfood.com, under the Evidence-Based Nutrition tab.

These fascinating stats only graze the surface. Basically, research suggests that nutrition can either help treat or help significantly reduce the risk of developing the following conditions:

- Heart disease
- Stroke
- Diabetes
- Inflammation
- Rheumatoid arthritis
- Fibromyalgia
- Distention and bloating
- IBS and IBD
- Leaky gut
- Headaches and migraines
- Heartburn and GERD
- Diarrhea, constipation, gas, cramps, and other stomach pains,
- Fatigue and decreased energy
- Frequent colds and illnesses
- Alzheimer's and dementia
- ADHD, hyperactivity, and general childhood behavior issues
- Cancer
- Mucus drainage and phlegm
- Seasonal allergies and asthma
- Brain function—lack of focus and attention and memory problems
- Joint pain
- Hormone imbalance
- Mood disorders—depression, anxiety, stress, schizophrenia, and bipolar
- Acne and aging skin
- Insomnia
- Inability to lose weight

- Small intestine bacteria overgrowth
- Autism
- Crohn's disease
- Lupus
- Ucerative colitis
- Celiac disease
- Multiple sclerosis
- Parkinson's

Inversely, diets high in ultra-processed foods—fried foods, refined sugars, sodas, processed meats, sugary pastries, red meats, beer, and vegetable oil—increase your risk of many of the same diseases and conditions.[40]

If you are feeling overwhelmed and wonder how you are ever going to remember everything you should be eating, don't worry. I included everything you need in this book: a checklist of all the foods you want to aim for each week and my Nourishing Meal Builder Chart.

Discussion Questions

1. Sometimes something becomes so normal that we forget how miraculous it is. Have you ever thought of food as a miracle? What are other everyday miracles of the earth and in life that we tend to take for granted? Close your eyes and silently take the time to thank God for these everyday miracles.

2. Genesis 1:29 (New International Version) says, "Then God said, 'I give you every seed-bearing plant on the face of the whole earth and every tree that has fruit with seed in it. They will be yours for food.'" And Psalms 136:25 (NIV) says, "He gives food to every creature. His love endures forever." Read these verses and discuss how they relate to the lesson above.

Weekly Challenge

Fruits and vegetables are powerhouses! They contain a multitude of antioxidants and filling fiber! This week's challenge is to eat a fruit or vegetable during every meal.

Discuss Last Week's Challenge

Last week, you were challenged to do a mini pause and prayer before speaking, whether in person, in a text, on the phone, in an email, or on social media. Discuss your observations and experiences. Did you seem to have more self-control? Were you more open and loving in your conversations with others?

LESSON 5
Can Faith-Based Mindfulness and Nutrition Help Us Live a Healthier, Happier, More Purposeful Life?

Mindfulness can help with our moods, behaviors, and even our health! The benefits of mindfulness cannot be overstated. In fact, mindfulness techniques are so beneficial that some schools have started implementing mindfulness programs.[41] One review looked at the mindfulness programs at thirteen schools. Overall, the children in these mindfulness programs saw improvements in their cognitive performance and resilience to stress. Although more research is needed, and the significance of the results varies between programs, current research indicates that implementing mindfulness programs in schools may improve social behaviors, mood, stress levels, and even academic performance and test scores. Schools are even reporting fewer suspensions, detentions, violent incidences, disciplinary visits to the principal's office, bullying, and classroom disruptions since incorporating mindfulness programs.[42]

If you think about it, these results make sense, don't they? Practicing mindfulness techniques can relieve stress and help us have better self-control. When we have less stress and learn to have more self-control, we tend to make better choices. Think about a time you were stressed. Did you let your emotions take over? Was it harder for you to act with love and kindness? I know I am less likely to choose love, patience, and compassion when I am boiling over with feelings of stress. Less ideal choices can sometimes cause even more stress, which brings us full circle. Furthermore, aren't we able to focus and learn better when our brains are calm versus when we're stressed? Mindfulness can help with stress and promote a more positive outlook on life. Less stress and more positivity promote better health. It's all beautifully related.

So you can see how mindfulness activities can be so impactful. Of course, for me, the most profound impact happens when I combine faith and mindfulness.

Remember, one aspect of mindfulness is focusing on being present, but with faith-based mindfulness, you are focusing on how God is present with you in that very moment. While focusing on God's presence, you get to notice all the gifts from God and the beautiful little things in God's world. This is why mindful living—and mindful eating since it's a part of mindful living—can help you live your healthiest, happiest, most purposeful life. I know, these are big words but hear me out. What do you want your life to look like? What about your children's lives? Are there things you would change? What does *your* healthiest, happiest, and most meaningful life look like? These are some of life's biggest questions. How do we attempt to answer them?

I am a list person, so when I consider these questions, my immediate impulse is to make a list:

1.   My greatest desire is to glorify God in all that I do. I want to show God's love through kindness and giving. My prayer is that I listen for God's guidance in every situation

because when I listen to God, amazing things happen, and I want to be *amazed*!

2. I wish to have a peaceful and positive life and a grateful attitude. I want to enjoy the little moments by taking the time to notice God's world and soak it up!

3. We humans seem to have a natural desire to work and create. We want to have meaning and purpose in our lives. This is true for me too. In my ideal life, I want to learn, grow, and work. I want to create something new and, at least in some small way, make the world better. I want to challenge my mind through reading and learning from God and others, and I want to challenge my body through physical activity.

4. Just as I desire to work, grow, and be challenged, I equally want to have time to rest, relax, and play. Sometimes, finding the time to relax is the most difficult challenge in life, yet it's so important for our health and our ability to serve God and others.

We may all have different wishes and desires, but when we break them down, I'm guessing that for people of faith, this list is at the heart of most of our desires. But how do we become this person and live this healthy, happy, more purposeful life? Faith-based mindfulness helps me fulfill that list like nothing else. Here is how my life has been transformed through faith-based mindfulness:

- I listen to God more, which helps me make better choices. I'm not letting negative emotions take control of my actions—at least, not as often, anyway.
- I am more at peace and comforted because I am noticing God is with me everywhere.
- I get to have more "goosebump moments" because when I intentionally focus on God in the present moment, I actually see what God is doing in my life and the lives of those around me. By focusing on God in the present

moment, I get to experience the feeling of amazement more often. Remember, I want to be *amazed*! Don't we all want to be beautifully amazed?

Do you see how all these benefits relate back to the goals I had listed above?

The Benefits of Faith-Based Mindful Eating

When you mindfully eat, you get to experience all the benefits of faith-based mindfulness. Mindful eating gives us the opportunity to focus on God's presence, feel gratitude for His gift of food, and rest our brains. We get to have mini mindfulness moments with God every time we eat!

God is guiding us through every aspect of life, including eating. In fact, God built a guide into our bodies. When we listen to the signals in our bodies, we stop eating when our bodies are nourished, and when we eat until our bodies tell us we are satisfied, we tend to naturally fall into the size that is healthiest for us. When we focus on what God's nourishing food can do for our bodies, we feel like celebrating every time we get the opportunity to eat nutrient-rich foods. Because we are thankful for healthy foods, we start eating healthier! Faith-based mindful eating helps us live healthier, less stressful lives.

How Does Nutrition Help Us Live Our Healthiest, Happiest, Most Purposeful Life?

Eating nourishing foods from God's earth feeds my mind, body, and soul so I can feel my best and have the energy to seize the day, which helps me live out the goals of my life I listed earlier.

Nourishing foods:

- Promote health and provide energy to serve God and others.
- Fuel our minds so we can learn and grow.

- Promote a positive mood. Although we should try to show kindness no matter what is going on in our lives, spreading kindness is so much easier when we aren't hurting inside. This is 100 percent true for me. Food can truly have an impact on how we feel, think, and act.
- Help our minds stay sharp, provide energy, and promote a positive mood, all of which are beneficial in regards to living our healthiest, happiest, most purposeful life.

Our bodies are not made to work all on their own. God provided what we need to survive and thrive. Such delicious food comes straight from the earth! In my opinion, this is why we humans need to do a better job getting food—this amazing gift from God—to our brothers and sisters all over the world.

Nutrition and Our Actions

I have learned to judge people less and less based on their actions. Maybe they had a hard day; maybe they experienced hardships I can't even imagine; maybe they have chemical imbalances or medical conditions and don't have control over how they are feeling or acting; or maybe they are just "hangry" in more ways than one. Have you heard of the term "hangry"? It refers to someone who is acting angry because they are hungry. I know I get this way, and my children certainly get this way when their blood sugar levels are too low. But I think we can still be hangry even when our stomachs are full if our bodies aren't getting all the nutrients they need. For example, maybe someone is having difficulty controlling their actions or mood because their brain is hungry for nutrients that promote optimal cognitive function and mood. Maybe they are in pain due to inflammation; thus, their body is "hangry" for anti-inflammatory foods. Pain, both emotionally and physically, can cause us to lash out at others. Being intentional or mindful about eating foods that nourish the mind, body, and soul can help with all types of "hanger." Nutrient deficiencies can cause mood swings, stress, and even depression—all of which can negatively affect the way we interact with others.

Discussion Questions

1. What does *your* healthiest, happiest, most meaningful life look like?
2. How might faith-based mindfulness help you live the life you want to live?
3. Similarly, how might nutrition help you live the life you want to live?
4. Psalms 46:10 (NIV) says, "Be still, and know that I am God." This is one of my favorite mindfulness Bible verses. What does this verse mean to you, and how does it relate to the mindful pause and slowing down?

    Note: I use the NIV translation for this verse because I like the images that come to my mind when I read, "Be still." I see someone frantically trying to get everything done. I see them hurrying from one job or chore to another. I see someone hastily trying to solve all life's problems on their own. I see their mind jumping from one thought to another or running down their never-ending to-do list over and over. Neither their body nor their mind can be still. Then God says, "Be still," and the person just stops. Then, in my mind's eye, I see relaxation and calmness overtake them as they come to acknowledge that God is God! So why worry? God's got this! This person I picture is me. Can you picture yourself in this scenario?
5. How can faith-based mindfulness and nutrition help us exhibit the characteristics described in Galatians 5:22–23 (NIV) (love, joy, peace, patience, kindness, goodness, faithfulness, gentleness, and self-control)?

Weekly Challenge

For this week's challenge, donate some nourishing food to a local food bank, shelter, friend, or family member who could use some extra love.

Discuss Last Week's Challenge

For last week's challenge, I asked you to eat a fruit or vegetable during every meal. What were your observations? Did you notice any differences in the way your mind or body felt?

PART 2
PUTTING IT INTO PRACTICE
(THE *HOW*)

LESSON 6
A Step-by-Step Guide to Faith-Based Mindful Eating

U p until now, the lessons have been mostly about the *why*. Remember, faith-based mindful eating can help us enjoy food more, which is a huge part of life; it also helps us cope with stress, promotes gut health (which reduces the risk and symptoms of many chronic conditions), and helps with weight loss when needed. Faith-based mindful eating also gives us the opportunity to draw closer to God, feel His presence, and appreciate His gift of food. But *how* do we go about incorporating mindful eating into our lives?

The next few lessons will go into actual faith-based mindfulness and nutrition techniques and strategies you can implement into your life.

Materials needed: a snack and water for each person in the class or for yourself if you are doing this study at home.

Step 1: Preparing Your Food

When preparing food, avoid mindlessly nibbling while you're cooking. Focus on the joy of cooking. For example, while sautéing vegetables, notice the steam, the smells, and the sound of the sizzle. Cooking will be more enjoyable and less stressful if you appreciate all the sights, sounds, and smells involved in the process.

Step 2: Plating Your Food

Make this process fun as well. Plate the food so it looks attractive to you. Hint: when you put too much on your plate, your plate doesn't look as nice as when you use less food. We eat with all our senses, including our vision, so how the plate looks is just as important for our eating experience as how the food tastes. When we pause to look at our plates before eating, we may feel more gratitude when we see an array of beautiful colors and textures.

When plating your food, be conscious of how much you are plating. *Pause* and ask yourself, "Is this a reasonable amount of food to nourish my body without making me feel overly full?" When we are overly full, we have eaten past what our bodies need. Plus, being overly full is unpleasant. After overeating, you might feel tired, sluggish, and bloated. Your stomach will feel uncomfortable, and you may even feel like you can't get a full breath. Think about a healthy, nourishing, and satisfying plate versus an over-the-top plate. How does your plate compare?

An overly full plate leaves little "white space." The different elements of your meal are on top of each other and might even be overtaking the edge of the plate. The food may also be piled high. If you turn another plate upside down and use it as a lid, and the rims of the plates don't come close to touching each other, then your food may be piled higher than you need. Remember that you don't need to overfill your plate because you can always go back for seconds if you notice you are still hungry.

Step 3: Eating Your Food

Sit down and eat. Before putting a bite in your mouth, *pause*. Really notice the food—its colors and textures—and think about how this food is going to benefit your body. When we think about how every bite of food affects us, we start to celebrate the opportunity to eat nutrient-rich ingredients. Instead of saying, "I need to" or "I have to" eat broccoli, we can start thinking, "I *get* to eat that broccoli." Pausing and thinking about the benefits helps personalize nutrition knowledge—you can look up the benefits of each food in Appendix A. In fact, when you are eating at home, you may want to look up the benefits of the foods you are eating before you take your first bite. You can then pause and thank God for each of the benefits before and during your eating experience.

Think of this moment as a time to focus on God's presence and feel grateful. Say a prayer before you begin eating. Thank God for this time to enjoy your food. By taking these steps, you are giving yourself a chance to more fully appreciate your food, and you are opening your mind to listen for God's guidance and feel His presence. Feeling God's presence is such a comfort, and we want to take every opportunity to experience this amazing feeling.

Before I pray over my food, I think about 1 Corinthians 10:31 (NIV), which says, "So whether you eat or drink or whatever you do, do it all for the glory of God." When I do pray, it goes something like this: "God, thank you so much for this food. I am so thankful that, right now, I get to sit and enjoy the food you have given me. I want to eat for the glory of You, God."

After saying your prayer, enjoy your food and your time eating in God's presence.

Continue to do mini pauses throughout the meal by putting your fork down between each bite. Prepare the next bite after you have swallowed and taken a sip of your drink. Intentionally take a sip of your drink between each bite. During the meal, *pause* occasionally to notice if you are full and ask yourself questions, like "Am I full?" or "How does this bite taste?" or "Am I enjoying my food?" or "Am I hungry or emotionally eating?" Asking these questions helps you stay mindfully aware throughout the meal. Remember, you not only will enjoy your food more but also will be able to notice when you are full if you are mindful throughout your whole meal. You will be surprised at how full and satisfied you will be after consuming the appropriate amount of food for your body. The key is pausing before you put food into your mouth. Listen to your body.

Mindful Eating Example

It was a crisp, fall Saturday, but I was warm and cozy inside my home. I was wearing an oversized, comfy sweatshirt and leggings. I had just started a load of laundry, and my children were playing upstairs. Occasionally, I would hear a *thud* followed by laughter. My children had eaten a late breakfast and weren't hungry yet, but I could feel a slight emptiness in my stomach. My hunger was there, but I wasn't feeling overly hungry yet. In other words, it was a good time to eat. I had already prepared a rice bowl the night before, so I decided to heat it up in the microwave.

When the microwave dinged, I pulled the bowl out of the microwave and walked to the table. I could see the steam coming from my reheated brown rice as I put my bowl on the table and sat down. As I looked at the food, the sounds of the children faded into the background. I was hungry, and the aroma from the spices made me feel excited about what I was about to eat. But I didn't start yet. First, I paused and took a moment to notice this gift from God. As I paused, I looked down at my food. The green broccoli, brown rice and beans, and orange sweet potatoes reminded me of the colors of God's earth on a beautiful fall day. I was overwhelmed by the miracle of food. Our bodies and minds need certain things to thrive, and I thanked God for providing them. I thought about how the brown rice, beans, and broccoli were full of filling fiber and how I have the privilege to eat broccoli, which contains valuable antioxidants. These antioxidants were going to help me in so many ways. Antioxidants reduce the risk of chronic disease and mood disorders, promote brain function, and support the immune system. *Right now*, I thought, *I get to eat foods that offer protection against Alzheimer's and cancer.* I thought about how sulforaphane found in broccoli may reduce the risk of some cancers and even reduce the size and number of cancer cells by 50–70 percent, and I got excited about the opportunity to eat broccoli.[43] *Right now, I get to eat foods that help me feel full and satisfied and provide energy for me to take on the day.*

Now I was ready to take that first glorious bite. As I bit down, my mouth exploded with the flavors of fresh garlic and spices. I could feel the gritty earthiness of the brown rice, which was yet another reminder that I was eating food from God's beautiful earth. It tasted like sweet nourishment, as if my body was flourishing with each bite. I could feel the creaminess of the black beans as my mouth broke up the outer skin. I continued to pray with each bite, thanking God for all that God has given us to help us thrive—fiber, vitamins and minerals, antioxidants, and protein.

As I ate, I also enjoyed God's company. I told God that I wanted to glorify Him in all I did, including eating. I thanked God some more for providing the energy and nutrients I need to go into the world and spread His love.

To this day, I continue to mindfully eat, making a conscious decision to be present with God and my food. With each bite, the stress of the day just melts away. This is a chance to rest my body and decompress. I can feel myself relaxing in God's presence. After having this time to refresh, I feel ready to seize the rest of the day. I feel confident that God is with me, helping me through anything the day might bring. I feel inspired to show kindness. I have energy now that I'm nourished with everything my mind, body, and soul need to function at their best.

Mindful Eating Activity

Instead of questions for this section, I'm going to have you eat and enjoy a snack through mindful eating.

Directions:

- Each person will get a snack and some water. Wait until everyone is ready before eating together.
- Before eating, *pause*. Look at your food and silently pray.
- Take a slow bite of your food. Then sit back and notice the flavors, smells, and textures. Wait until you have finished the first bite before preparing the next. Many of us begin preparing our next bite while eating the first one. If we are busy scooping up our next bite, are we really taking the time to enjoy the food?
- After you have completely swallowed, clean your palate with water.
- Now, prepare your next bite and repeat the process.

Weekly Challenge

Try following the above steps to mindfully eat each meal this week.

Discuss Last Week's Challenge

Last week, I challenged you to donate nourishing food to a food bank, shelter, friend, or family member. Did you have a chance to do it? If so, talk about what you did. If not, think about who you might donate food to this week.

LESSON 7
What Does a Mindful Day Look Like?

Mindfulness is about being in the present moment. The past is gone, and the future has not happened, but the present is *here* and *now*.

Think about it.

What two things do we spend most of our time stressing over and worrying about? The mistakes we made in the past and the unknown future. How much less stress would we have if we learned to focus on the present moment? My guess is *a lot*!

Mindful eating is about focusing on eating and enjoying every bite. Mindful living is about focusing and enjoying whatever you are doing in that moment. Mindfulness is also about having a grateful approach to life. When we are mindfully living, we focus on the positive and the things we're thankful for in the present moment. For me, mindfulness is about focusing on God's presence in our lives at every moment and focusing on the beauty in God's world. Sounds simple, right? Yeah, I know. It is a lot easier said than done. Sometimes, we will still worry about the past and the future, but fortunately, mindfulness techniques can help us live in the present a little more often. So here it is: the faith-based mindfulness guide.

Pause, Breathe, and Pray Before, Well, *Everything*

Remember to pause. Take a moment to breathe and mindfully pray before entering a new environment and before eating.

Before entering a new place, I ask God to help me remember to show love and kindness in this current environment. I then thank God for being with me, and I pray that I hear and mindfully listen for God's guidance while I am in this place. I pray on the way to my kid's school, before entering the grocery store, before entering my friend's house, or on the way to a park. I pray before a family reunion or a meeting at work. God really is with us, communicating with us. We just need to stop and hear what He is saying. When I pause, I am more likely to speak and act the way God wants me to—with love. God finds ways to speak words of comfort as well. Praying before these situations gives us time to let God embrace us.

Another great place to pause and pray is at a red light. Instead of feeling impatient and bored while waiting for the light to change, try taking deep breaths and praying. Use the red light as a time to relax and be present. By doing this, we remember God is with us everywhere. By pausing, breathing, and praying, we can better focus on the moment and on God in every place. You will notice the joy in the mundane when you focus on the small treasures of each moment. You will also have a heightened experience if you focus on being present during fun, exciting times, and although you will still experience pain during sad or scary times, you can find comfort when you lean on God through prayer.

When I forget to pause and pray after waking up in the morning or going to bed at night, I notice the difference in my actions and behavior. I become moody and speak harshly to people, including my children. This act of pausing before everything really helps keep me calm and comforted, which causes me to react in a more loving way. Yes, I pause before meals, but pausing before every new situation is also crucial to my behavior, actions, and mood.

Use Your Senses to Focus on the People and the Place

Once you have entered a new environment, place, or building, the next step is to focus on the people around you and the place you are in. In other words, use your senses to be present in the moment instead of thinking about all the things you must do later. This is particularly important to me when I am with my children. Worrying about all I must do doesn't help me, and I actually end up missing out on beautiful moments with my kids. Why worry about things you can't do anything about at the moment?

I recently caught myself worrying instead of being present with one of my children. It was time to drop my child off at choir practice. When we arrived, no one was there yet, including the teacher. I was late for a meeting at work, but I had to wait on my daughter's teacher to arrive before I could leave. While I was impatiently waiting, my four-year-old daughter was just twirling around and giggling. I suddenly realized I was missing out on what was right in front of me: my daughter, living in the moment! Her dress swirled around her as she danced. Some of her hair had fallen out of her ponytail and looked as if it was floating as she twirled. I remembered how much I had loved twirling when I was young. Why was I not twirling too? To my daughter's delight, I joined her. That dizzy feeling you get when twirling was exhilarating.

At that moment, I stopped worrying and started twirling and giggling with my daughter. That moment of waiting ended up being a beautiful, special moment because I chose to focus on my daughter. I couldn't do anything about being late, so why should I worry?

Practice Gratitude—There Are Actual Exercises That Can Help!

When we approach life with a grateful attitude and look for the good in life, the benefits are endless. Research shows that gratitude practices have been associated with improved glycemic and asthma control, reduction in blood pressure, decreased stress and inflammation, and increased reports of happiness and overall well-being.[44] When we focus on the positive aspects of life, we tend to have more compassion and kindness for others; thus, the circle of positivity continues. Now the person you showed kindness to may leave feeling more grateful and positive. Now they will be more likely to pass it on.

I recently was on the receiving end of a kind gesture that motivated me to pass it on. I had just found a parking spot at the beach and was about to pay the meter for a ticket when a stranger approached.

She said, "Excuse me, are you about to pay for a ticket? I paid for one but have to leave, and I still have several hours left on my ticket. Would you like to have mine?"

She didn't have to take the time to ask a stranger if they needed a ticket, but she did.

Do you know what she said when I thanked her? She said, "Pay it forward."

I was determined to do just that, and I soon had my opportunity.

The next day, my family and I were standing in a long line at an amusement park in the heat. Behind us, a little boy, about four-years-old, was crying, "I'm hot, Mommy! I want water!"

We had a fan that also spritzed water, so, thinking of the kindness shown to me the day before, I decided to let the little boy hold the water fan for the remainder of the line. When he reached for the fan, his crying immediately stopped. He was happy for the rest of the wait, and I could tell his mom, who happened to be very pregnant, was happy too. I would have let him keep it, but his mom, filled with gratitude, insisted he return it before they jumped on the ride. We all experienced gratitude because of one stranger's act of kindness.

Do you know there are specific strategies you can implement that can help you have a more grateful attitude?

a. **Creating Opportunities for Quiet Time**

We all need to rest. We need time to clear our thoughts and feel the weight of responsibility lifted for a little while. When I take time to just relax in God's presence, it feels like a chance to completely be myself with the only One who loves me unconditionally. The problems of the world are gone for a moment. I am safe, free, and at peace. My favorite ways to experience quiet time with God is through prayer, reading— either the Bible or uplifting faith books—and journaling.

b. **Journaling Mindfully**

You can practice gratitude, focus on God's presence, and have quiet time all through mindful journaling. Keeping a journal has been a part of my life for years, but I truly saw the difference in my outlook on life when I focused on God and gratitude as I wrote. Sometimes, I found myself just venting and complaining. When I shifted to a journal focused on gratitude, I noticed I eventually started feeling the way I was writing. I realized my life was filled with so many gifts, and focusing on those gifts made me happier. It's okay to vent in your journals when you need to get something off of your chest. I still vent sometimes, but the focus of my journal is positive. The key is to mostly focus on the good. We can easily get into a complaining habit, which will only produce more negative feelings. Even when I vent, I try to include positive aspects and even compassion for the situation and individuals in the situation.

Things to Include in Your Mindful Journal:
- All the positive things about the day and what you are grateful for
- Written prayers or letters to God
- Any lessons you learned through either your life experiences, reading, or Bible studies

- Any questions you have about life
- "God Moment" stories
  - o These are stories about when you noticed God working in your life. One cool thing about taking the time to mindfully notice God's presence every day is that you, well, really notice God's presence regularly and see what He's doing in your life.
  - o Since I started mindfully taking the time to notice God in the present moment, I have had so many God moments. These are the moments I think I will remember forever, but as time passes, I find I can't remember the details as well. Before including these "God Moment" stories in my journal, I would remember something pretty cool happened, but I couldn't bring the vague memory to the surface in my mind. By including these "God Moment" stories in my journal, I solidify these events to my memory. So if I do forget them, I can look at my journal and experience the awe and wonder all over again.

Eat Mindfully and with Faith

As mentioned earlier, mindful eating is yet another time to pause and focus on God, feel grateful, and enjoy a peaceful experience. You can review faith-based mindful techniques in Lesson 5.

Discussion Questions

1. For a moment, take the time to pause and silently pray for the people in the room, even if it's just you. Thank God for them and ask God to help you be loving and kind to the people God has put into your life in this very moment. While you are pausing, take time to notice your surroundings. Is there something to be thankful for? The chair you are sitting in? The temperature-controlled room? The sound of the wind in the trees outside or the birds chirping?

2. What three things in your life are you thankful for right now?

3. Colossians 3:15 (NIV) says, "Let the peace of Christ rule in your hearts, since as members of one body you were called to peace. And be thankful." Philippians 4:6 (NIV) says, "Do not be anxious about anything, but in every situation, by prayer and petition, with thanksgiving, present your requests to God." And Colossians 4:2 (NIV) says, "Devote yourselves to prayer, being watchful and thankful." What do you think these Bible verses say about prayer, mindfulness, and thankfulness?

Weekly Challenge

For this week, try to spend some time writing what you are thankful for in a mindful journal.

Discussion of Last Week's Challenge

Last week's challenge was to mindfully eat your meals. What are some things you noticed about mindful eating? Did you enjoy your food and your time eating a meal with God? Did it help you feel less stress? Did it seem to help with portion control?

LESSON 8
How to Build a Nourishing Meal

Based on what we have learned in previous lessons, we can see just how impactful nutrition is to our minds, bodies, and souls, but the next question is, "What foods should I be eating?" Well, as mentioned earlier, I have spent years collecting nutrition research. I touched on some of the most fascinating stats from the research earlier, but to simplify the researchs here are the nutrients our body needs in order to thrive:

- Antioxidants like vitamin A, vitamin C, vitamin E, polyphenols, flavonoids, selenium, glutathione, and quercetin
- Vitamins and minerals like B vitamins, potassium, zinc, iron, magnesium, calcium, vitamin D, and vitamin K
- Fiber including beta-glucan
- Healthy fats including monounsaturated fats and omega-3s
- Prebiotics and probiotics
- Amino acids found in protein-rich foods
- Melatonin—found in cherries—and lycopene—another antioxidant found in red fruits

Okay, *now* how do we easily incorporate all these essential and beneficial nutrients into our diets? Fortunately, there's a general guide that will help us to, for the most part, get the foods that do all the amazing things I mentioned in Lesson 4.

And guess what? I have provided the guide in the following pages!

MEAL PLAN CHECKLIST

A HEALTHY DIET	NOTES
❑ Mostly plant-based	
❑ Whole grains: 2–3X/day Alternate whole grains to reduce the likelihood of developing a food sensitivity.	–Example grains include oats, quinoa, buckwheat, whole wheat, brown rice, wild rice.
❑ Vegetables: every meal	
❑ Leafy greens: 1X/day	
❑ Nuts/Seeds: 5X/week	–Example nuts/seeds include walnuts, almonds, pistachios, chia seeds, flax seeds, hemp seeds..
❑ Beans/Legumes: 4X/week	
❑ Poultry: 2X/week	
❑ Fish (Salmon): 2X/week	
❑ Fruit: every day	
❑ Berries: 2X/week	

MEAL PLAN CHECKLIST

A HEALTHY DIET	NOTES
❏ Probiotics: 4-5X/week (yogurt and cultured foods)	
❏ Include a variety of fresh spices in your meals	–Example spices include thyme, turmeric (and black pepper), rosemary, cinnamon, ginger, sage, garlic, cilantro.

EAT LESS OFTEN

- Refined sugar/refined grains
- Added sugar
- Fried foods
- Red meat
- Smoked meats
- Beer
- Heavily processed foods (ex: boxed pastries, hotdogs, bologna, luncheon meats—nitate & nitrite free are better choices—boxed foods with long ingredients list

In addition to this checklist, you may want to consider adding green tea, chamomile tea, dark chocolate, and nutritional yeast to your meals from time to time.

Cool, we know the general guidelines, but how do we turn that information into everyday meals?

I have another easy strategy for you. I call it the "Meal Builder." The Meal Builder is an easy way to put your meal-plan checklist into practice. At first, you may feel intimidated. Maybe you think you aren't good at cooking, or you wonder how you will put together a meal without a recipe. However, once you just try it a few times, you will see how easy it is. With the Meal Builder, you don't need to follow a bunch of recipes or take the time to plan meals every day. Simply pick foods from each category—a base, a protein, a few vegetables, and some sauces and seasonings—then, select your cooking method from the meal building table, and you have created a recipe. It's so easy and fun! You will not believe the delicious meals you can create!

The best way to learn how to build a meal is to follow the meal-building steps found below in the Meal Builder table.

Now, you may ask, "But what about when I am eating out?" If you are dining out, think about your checklist as you pick your meals. Be mindful of your choices and how they will make you feel.

THE MEAL BUILDER
CHOOSE FROM EACH BLOCK TO BUILD A MEAL

BASE (CHOOSE 1)

• Oats	• Mashed beans	• Whole grain pizza crust
• Chickpea pasta	• Kasha	• Whole grain bread,
• Zoodles	• Pamini pasta	Sub rolls, buns, english
• Palmini	• Cauliflower pizza	muffins, etc.
• Black bean pasta	Crust	• Lettuce, kale, spinach for
• Quinoa	• Cauliflower knochi	a salad
• Whole grain pasta	• Spaghetti squash	• Baked chips made with
• Cauliflower rice/	• Soba noodles	whole grains, flaxseed,
mashed	• Spring roll wrap	black beans, or quinoa
• Lentil pasta	• Konjac noodles	(Find the healthiest chips
• Cauliflower or	• Lettuce leaves as	and crackers on my blog)
Broccoli tots (I like	a wrap	• Crackers made from
Green Giant)	• Cloud bread (find	whole grain, flaxseed, chia
	the recipe on	seeds, etc.)
	my blog)	• Whole grain wraps to
	• Brown rice	make wraps, pizza, tacos,
		or quesadillas (I like Ole'
		Xtreme High Fiber)

PROTEIN (CHOOSE 1)

• Salmon fillet	• Nuts and seeds (like	• Ground turkey
• Canned salmon or	almonds, walnuts,	• Frozen veggie burgers
salmon packets	pistaccios, pumpkin	(I like Amy's California
• Eggs	seeds, chia seeds,	Veggie)
• Grilled fish	flaxseeds, hemp	• No nitrate/nitrite added
• Birdseye steam	seeds, etc.)	Turkey Slices
fresh protein	• Beans, canned or	• No nitrate/nitrite added
blends	frozen (any variety:	chicken sausage (I like
• Canned	cannanelli, kidney,	Applegate)
chickpeas	black eyed, black, etc.)	• Nutritional yeast
• Canned tuna or	• Grilled chicken	
tuna packets/	• Ground chicken	
pouches		

THE MEAL BUILDER
CHOOSE FROM EACH BLOCK TO BUILD A MEAL

VEGETABLE (CHOOSE 3 OR MORE)

• Zucchini	• Asparagus	• Brussels sprouts
• Broccoli	• Cherry tomatoes	• Frozen vegetable mixes
• Corn	• Green beans	• Beans (any variety)
• Onion	• Peas	• Peppers (any variety)
• Kimchi (I like Mother in Law brand)	• Sun-dried tomatoes	• Sweet potatoes
• Celery	• Jar of capers	• Mushrooms
• Sauerkraut (I like Farmhouse Culture brand)	• Carrots	• Artichokes
• Tomato	• Slaw packs (broccoli, cabbage, kale, etc.)	• Fermented pickles
• Cucumber	• Cabbage	• Salsa
• Kale	• Cauliflower	• Pico del gallo
• Spinach	• Squash (any variety)	• Roasted red peppers
	• Avocados	

SUPER ADD-INS (OPTIONAL)

- Flaxseeds
- Hemp seeds
- Chia seeds

CHEESES (OPTIONAL)

- Parmesan
- Mozzarella
- Cheddar
- Goat
- Ricotta
- Nutritional yeast (cheese substitute)

THE MEAL BUILDER
SEASONING AND SAUCE COMBINATIONS
(CHOOSE 2 OR MORE FROM 1 BLOCK)

ASIAN INSPIRED

- Teriyaki sauce (Primal Kitchen) or soy sauce + choices below:
  - Garlic
  - Sesame oil
  - Salt
  - Black pepper
  - Honey + ketchup (I like Primal Kitchen brand)
  - Siracha sauce
  - Mirin
  - For creamy sauce: cream cheese, yogurt, or a can of cream soup
  - Asian vinaigrette
  - Chicken/vegetable broth

CURRY

- Tomato sauce + Honey + seasonings below:
  - Coriander
  - Cumin
  - Tumeric and black pepper
  - Garlic
  - For creamy sauce: cream cheese, yogurt (add after cooking), or a can of cream soup
  - Ginger
  - Cayenne pepper
  - Mustard

DRESSINGS AND VINAGARETTES

- Honey + vinegar
- Balsamic or cider vinegar
- Black pepper
- Chicken/vegetable broth
- Onion powder mix
- Extra virgin olive oil

- White pepper
- Italian dressing (I like Primal Kitchen)
- For creamy sauce: cream cheese, yogurt (add after cooking), or a can of cream soup

THE MEAL BUILDER
SEASONING AND SAUCE COMBINATIONS

(CHOOSE 2 OR MORE FROM 1 BLOCK)

ITALIAN

- Montreal seasoning
- Tomato sauce (I like Primal Kitchen)
- Italian seasoning
- Parsley
- Oregano
- Garlic
- Black pepper
- Salt
- Honey
- Basil
- Sage
- Tomato soup can
- For creamy sauce: cream cheese, yogurt (add after cooking), or a can of cream soup)
- White pepper
- Extra virgin olive oil

BBQ

- Montreal seasoning
- BBQ sauce (I like Primal Kitchen)
- White pepper
- Turmeric and black pepper
- Garlic
- Worcestershire sauce

CHILI

- Montreal seasoning
- Chili seasoning
- Chicken broth
- Cream cheese (For a creamy sauce)
- Salt
- Yogurt (add after cooking to preserve live bacteria)
- White pepper, black pepper, or cayenne pepper
- Garlic
- Worcestershire sauce

THE MEAL BUILDER
SEASONING AND SAUCE COMBINATIONS
(CHOOSE 2 OR MORE FROM 1 BLOCK)

MARINATE INSPIRED	KICKIN' "SAUSAGE"
• Italian dressing/vinigarette • White wine sauce • Garlic • Capers • Lemon juice • Parsley • Chicken broth • Vegetable broth • Black pepper • Salt • Cider/balsamic vinegar • Extra virgin olive oil	• Fennel seeds • Garlic • Paprika • Black pepper • Salt • White pepper • BBQ sauce • Worcestershire sauce • For creamy sauce: cream cheese, yogurt (add after cooking), or a can of cream soup

SOUTHWEST INSPIRED	
• Chipotle adobe sauce • Chicken broth/vegetable broth • Taco seasoning (I like Simply Organic) • Garlic • Paprika • Salt • Lime juice • Lemon juice • For creamy sauce: cream cheese, yogurt (add after cooking), sour cream, or a can of cream soup	• Tomato sauce • Extra virgin olive oil • Avocado oil • Cilantro • White pepper • Cayenne pepper • Sriracha sauce • Cumin

THE MEAL BUILDER
SEASONING AND SAUCE COMBINATIONS
(CHOOSE 2 OR MORE FROM 1 BLOCK)

GET CREATIVE

• Hot sauce	• White pepper
• Montreal seasoning	• Turmeric and black pepper
• White wine	• For creamy sauce: cream cheese,
• Garlic	yogurt (add after cooking), sour
• Salt	cream, or a can of cream soup
• Pepper	• Extra virgin olive oil
• Chicken/vegetable broth	• Salad dressings made with less sugar
• Onion soup mix	and simple ingredients (I like Primal
• Ranch packets	Kitchen)
• Worcestershire	• Everything but the bagel seasoning
• Paprika	
• BBQ sauce	

PESTO
CHOOSE ALL ON THE LIST, MIX IN A FOOD PROCESSOR
SAUTE WITH INGREDIENTS FROM OTHER CARDS

• Basil	• Garlic
• Leafy Green	• Olive Oil
• Pine Nuts or other nuts	• Black Pepper
• Parmesan Cheese	• Salt

THE MEAL BUILDER
SEASONING AND SAUCE COMBINATIONS
(CHOOSE 2 OR MORE FROM 1 BLOCK)

ALFREDO
USE THE INGREDIENTS BELOW TO MAKE A HEALTHY ALFREDO OR SIMPLY USE PRIMAL KITCHEN'S ALFREDO SAUCE

- Parmesan
- Garlic
- Salt
- Black pepper
- Cream cheese
- Vegetable broth
- Milk (I like 1% Omega-3 Milk)

SIGNATURE
MIX ALL THE INGREDIENTS BELOW TO MAKE A SIGNATURE SAUCE

- Horseradish
- Avocado or olive oil mayo (I like Primal Kitchen)
- Lemon juice
- BBQ sauce (I like Primal Kitchen)
- Honey
- Sriracha sauce

THE MEAL BUILDER

SEASONING AND SAUCE COMBINATIONS

(CHOOSE 2 OR MORE FROM 1 BLOCK)

KEEP IT SIMPLE

A note on sauces: choosing healthy condiments, sauces, and dressings can be overwhelming. You want your sauces and condiments to provide nourishment, and yet sometimes you just don't want to make a sauce from scratch. This is why I love the Primal Kitchen brand. These dressings, condiments, and sauces have no sugar added and use simple, whole ingredients. So when I want to keep things simple, I just pick a base, pick my vegetables, pick a protein, and add a Primal Kitchen sauce or dressing. Bam! My recipe is done!

THE MEAL BUILDER

CHOOSE A COOKING METHOD (1 OR MORE)

Sauté

Bake
* Perfect for mixed and layered casseroles

Slow Cooker

Pressure Cooker

THE MEAL BUILDER

CHOOSE A COOKING METHOD (1 OR MORE)

Sandwich, Wrap, Lettuce Wrap

Dip with Chips/Crackers

Salad

"Meat"Ball/Patty

*Just add egg or flaxseed and water to chosen ingredients and form a ball or patty; bake or sauté

THE MEAL BUILDER

CHOOSE A COOKING METHOD (1 OR MORE)

Egg Muffin Cup

Add eggs and ingredients of your choice
to a muffin cup and bake

Below are simple steps to building your nourishing meals.

- **Step 1:** grocery shop using the Meal Builder chart. You don't need to have any specific meals in mind, but you can if you want. You simply need to pick a variety of bases, proteins, vegetables, sauces, and seasonings. Also, be sure to include fruits and snacks. Use the "Is It Healthy?" table when you select your snacks. Now, you will have everything you need to make a healthy meal on the fly.
- **Step 2:** pick your base from the Base list.
- **Step 3:** pick a protein or two from the Protein list.
- **Step 4:** pick as many vegetables as you want from the Vegetable list.
- **Step 5:** pick the seasoning and sauces from one of the Seasoning and Sauces lists. **NOTE:** In the blocks on the previous pages, I grouped seasonings and sauces together so that no matter which combination of sauces you pick on the list, they will always taste fantastic together—preferences vary, of course! If you desire a "soupier" or stew-type meal, add more broth and sauces, such as tomato sauce. If you want a creamier sauce, add the yogurt or cream soups. For a sandwich, you may want to use less "soupy" ingredients. Seasoning and oils work great together for sautéed vegetables and proteins.
- **Step 6:** pick a healthy addition and an occasional cheese, if desired.
- **Step 7:** pick a cooking method from one block.

Here are a few notes about each type of cooking method and how to use them as part of the meal builder.

Cook your ground meat first. Then you can add the meat to your other ingredients and bake, sauté, slow cook, etc.

How to brown ground meat:

1. If you are using extra-lean ground meat, spray the skillet with non-stick cooking spray.
2. Heat the spray over medium-high heat.
3. Once the pan is hot, add the meat.
4. Use a spatula to break up the meat into smaller pieces.
5. Spread the meat evenly in the pan. Then let the meat cook for about five minutes.
6. Sprinkle meat with the seasonings of your choice.
7. Stir the meat until you no longer see any pink.
8. Drain the fat from the meat. Never put the drained fat in the sink drain. Discard the excess fat in a tin can or glass jar. Place the container in the refrigerator until the fat has cooled. Once the fat has cooled, place the fat in a sealed container and discard it. Pouring fat into the drain can cause clogging. Pouring hot fat directly into the trash could cause the trash bags to melt, creating a mess.
9. Note: cook the brown rice or whole-grain pasta separately per direction on the package before combining it in a casserole dish or pan. You can substitute half the water with broth to add flavor.

Slow cooker instructions:

- Defrosted uncooked chicken can go straight into the slow cooker.
- Do not cook rice or pasta in the slow cooker with the other ingredients. Add the cooked rice or pasta to your slow-cooking food after your food is done.

Baking instructions:

- When baking a casserole, make sure your meal contains some kind of "wet" ingredient in the casserole dish, such as tomato sauce, broth, creamy sauce, yogurt, etc. Remember to brown ground meat before cooking it in the oven. Chicken can go in the oven uncooked.
- Temperature varies, but 375 degrees is a good start. Cover casserole dishes with tinfoil while they are is baking. Check every ten minutes to see if the food is done.
- You can bake less "wet" foods on a sheet pan uncovered but remember that different foods will cook at different times. For example, chicken will take longer than fish. Basting your food with oil will help the food brown. Check your food often. Vegetables can take anywhere between ten to fifty minutes at 400 degrees. Fish will only take around ten minutes at four hundred degrees. Chicken will vary depending on the size but can take around twenty to forty-five minutes at 400 degrees. The key is to keep checking your food often.

Dips:

- Ingredients should be chopped or blended into smaller pieces when used in a dip. Make sure to add a "wet," creamy ingredient to dips. Make sure all food that must be cooked is cooked thoroughly.
- Crackers, chips, or even raw vegetables can be the base for dips.

Pressure cooker instructions:

- Add the food and liquid in the pressure cooker pot.
- Close the lid and set the valve to the correct setting. You will have to look up a time chart for the ingredients you are cooking. You can find this online or in the packet that comes with many pressure cookers.

- Wait for pressure to build up in the pot.
- Start the pressure cooker.
- When the food is finished cooking and the timer has stopped, release the pressure.

Sautéing instructions:

- Sauté meat and vegetables separately.
- Heat the pan on medium-high heat before adding the oil.
- Add just enough oil to coat the bottom of the pan.
- Add bite-size pieces of your food to the pan. Don't overfill. You should have one layer of food on the pan.
- Turn the food with a fork or spatula when it is lightly browned or crunchy on one side. Overcooked vegetables can become mushy.

Wraps, salads, and sandwiches:

- For wraps, salads, or sandwiches, the base would be either a tortilla, lettuce, or some type of bread.
- You can add ingredients that are edible when raw or ingredients that need to be cooked before eaten. **Note:** if you are not sure what to do when cooking, look up "how to" steps for different cooking methods and foods online. Experiment and have fun! Soon, you will feel like a professional chef.

IS IT HEALTHY?

❑ Minimal refined grains

❑ A whole food is listed as the first ingredient

❑ Minimal added sugar (no added sugar is best!).

❑ Simple ingredients list

❑ No trans fats

❑ Contains beneficial nutrients (vitamins, minerals, fiber, antioxidants, omega-3s, probiotics, etc.)

When choosing which brand of seasoning and sauces to use, follow the "Is It Healthy?" chart on the previous page. This chart is a helpful reference for choosing packaged snacks as well.

Discussion Questions

Practice building an imaginary meal. What base would you choose? What protein and vegetables? Now what seasonings and sauces would you combine? Now pick your cooking method. Practice this several times.

Weekly Challenge

1. Try to build a meal using the foods recommended in the "Meal Plan Checklist" and the "Meal Builder" technique. Remember to pause and pray before you mindfully enjoy your meal.
2. As you prepare your meals, slow down and enjoy the adventure. Take the time to praise God during the cooking process.
3. First Corinthians 10:31 (NIV) says, "So, whether you eat or drink, or whatever you do, do all to the glory of God."

Discuss Last Week's Challenge

Last week's challenge was to write down what you were thankful for. Look over what you wrote down and reflect.

PART 3
LESSONS FROM GOOSEBUMP STORIES AND BEING MINDFULLY AWARE OF GOD'S PRESENCE

When I incorporated faith-based mindfulness into my life, I started noticing God's presence more often. In this next section, I share some of the "goosebump stories" I have had in my life. Some of them seemingly came out of nowhere while others came after prayer. God is with us always, whether we are mindful or not, but you might notice many of the stories occur after I incorporated mindfulness. This doesn't mean God was not doing things in my life before; rather, it means I finally slowed down enough to really notice.

LESSON 9
God Loves Us

I first realized just how much God loved me, and all of us, when I was in middle school. Here is my story.

It was the first day of middle school. I felt all grown up and ready to meet new people. After much deliberation on what outfit to wear, I had carefully decided on a pink V-neck shirt and a pair of jean shorts that had a pink ruffle on the bottom. The first few weeks of sixth grade went okay. I was making new friends, but I became particularly close with two girls—let's call them Cindy and Addi. I don't remember exactly how we connected, but I do remember they were fun and relatable. We went over to each other's houses and talked on the phone every night. We got along great, which was why I was confused when, one day, Cindy decided to make me the outcast. To this day, I still don't know what exactly happened. Maybe I did something I wasn't even aware of, or maybe it was because I started gaining weight and getting pimples. Maybe I was just too awkward and dorky. But one thing was clear: she made it her mission to let everyone know that I was "unfriendable."

I do have a theory, though. As a sixth-grader, you often feel like you need to put others down to make yourself look better. Seriously, sixth grade is brutal. Someone must be the outcast, and you have to make sure it is someone other than you. If you can put down someone else, then people will pay attention to you. If you want to be cool, you must show how utterly uncool someone else is. Someone must be the loser or outcast so someone else can be the winner. At least, that's what you think when you are in middle school.

The Outcast

It was a normal school day, but during class, I noticed Cindy seemed a little standoffish. I just brushed it off. The next few days, the ignoring seemed to get worse and worse. And then one day, during gym class, Cindy made it very clear she didn't want to be friends with me anymore. We were practicing lay-ups, and Cindy had just made a shot. As she walked back to the line, I held out my hand for her to give me a high five. She would not even look at me. She just walked right past me, ran straight to another girl, and started giggling.

Ignoring me was just the beginning. She then began spreading rumors about me. I am also not sure what the rumors were. I would just hear different things from different people. Shortly after the rumors had spread, I saw a group of girls talking before class. As I approached, one girl whispered, "Here comes Lacy. Everyone turn your back." Then, when I tried to greet the group, the girls, including Cindy, huddled together in a circle with their backs to me and did not speak.

Worst Lunch Ever

On the worst day, a girl I didn't know and I walked to the lunch table where we usually sat, but no one was there. I know you are wondering how I didn't know the other girl if we usually sat at the same table, but the table was long, and she often sat at the other end of it. We both started to sit down at our ends of the table, but then we noticed a few of the girls we usually sat with standing near a table on the other side of the vast lunchroom. This girl and I walked over to them and asked, "Are we were sitting over here today?"

One of them replied nonchalantly, "No, we are sitting over there. Go save us a seat."

The other girl and I sat at the other table, saving seats for our friends, but our friends never came to the table. The two of us were sitting at a huge table all by ourselves. You can imagine what that does to an eleven-year-old girl's reputation. The other girl looked visibly upset when she came to the realization that we had been abandoned. She muttered something I didn't catch under her breath as she forcefully stood up to leave. I sometimes wonder if she was just collateral damage because the girls were actually just trying to get away from me. Now alone, I decided to move to another table with a different set of girls. Then the girls at that table thought it would be funny to throw my lunch on the ground. My lunch was ruined.

Alone

These kinds of incidences went on throughout sixth grade. I felt so alone, like I didn't have a single friend in the world. I hated going to school. In fact, I dreaded it!

Although my parents were amazing—something I am so grateful for—I didn't feel happy at home either because going home meant night was coming, and I would have to try to sleep. But I couldn't sleep at all. I was so lonely, and the dark made me feel even more alone. I would lie there absolutely terrified. My heart felt like it was in my throat. It felt like I was drowning in despair. I tried to hide my fear of the dark from my parents because I didn't want them to feel sorry for me or feel like their daughter was a loser.

Is God Actually Real?

I began thinking about things that I had never thought about before. I started wondering if God really existed, and if so, why was God letting the other kids be so mean to me? My simple eleven-year-old mind thought if I was mostly good, God wouldn't let me experience such misery. Maybe God didn't love me as much as everyone at church said. Or worse, maybe God wasn't even real.

Why should I even believe in God? Just because my parents said so? I would think.

I had never really given God much thought before. Sure, I went to church, knew the story, and even accepted it as true, but I never truly understood.

I Decided to Pray ...

With these thoughts running through my head, I decided to pray and ask God point-blank, "God, if You are real, show me a sign."

Within the same week, while walking home from school on the road I took every day, I saw a tree shaped like a cross. I had never seen it before even though I had taken that path every day for a year.

... And *This* Happened!

Shortly after, I was lying on the couch one night and watching TV with my parents. As usual, I was feeling terribly sad and alone, dreading the inevitable bedtime, when out of the blue, I felt God tell me, "I love you." I wasn't watching anything spiritual or thinking about God. The words just came out of nowhere. I didn't hear a voice; I felt the words being said to me. At that moment, a weird warmth came over me, and I felt an indescribable joy, greater than I had ever felt before. I knew that even though I did not feel loved at school, I was not alone. Someone who loved me was with me all the time, even at school. I wasn't alone at night while I slept in my room either.

God was telling me He loved me. I wasn't alone ever.

I knew the words had come from God because my life changed after that. Suddenly, I didn't dread going to school or to my room at night. I didn't care what people said anymore because an almighty being loved me. Everything else seemed trivial. I truly didn't care what people thought of me anymore, and somehow, I almost instantly found new friends. The ignoring, teasing, and rumors stopped ... or, at least, I didn't notice them anymore. I loved going to church. I started having fun at youth group. Oh, and I slept. Beautiful, wonderful sleep! I loved going to my room because it was a chance for me to be alone with God. I would often pray myself to sleep. This was truly the beginning of my new life with God.

Now, I realize that the year of being teased and bullied was a miracle. Although I was not and am not even close to perfect, after that experience, I was more aware of my actions toward others all throughout middle school and high school. I was careful not to make fun of and be cruel to others because I knew what that felt like. I know I failed sometimes because I was still a middle-school girl. Nonetheless, I am thankful that God showed me how much it hurt to be picked on or bullied so I could be more aware of how my actions can affect people.

God Loves *You* Too

I couldn't believe the love God felt for me. It was so strong! And you know what? God feels that way about you too. God loves you so unbelievably much. You are not alone.

Discussion Questions

1. What does it mean to bully someone? Have you ever experienced bullying? Does bullying happen among adults as well? In what way (if any) could the mindfulness techniques help stop us from bullying others?
2. Have you ever had something good come from a painful experience? How did a painful experience help you grow closer to God or grow as a person?
3. What does my story say about God's love for us?
4. Matthew 7:12 (ESV) says, "So whatever you wish that others would do to you, do also to them, for this is the Law and the Prophets." What does this Bible verse mean to you? How would living our lives like this Bible verse prevent us from bullying others?

Weekly Challenge

Do the opposite of bullying others this week. Build someone up through words of encouragement. Make a conscience effort to encourage someone either in person or on social media, or both!

Discuss Last Week's Challenge

Last week, you were challenged to build a meal using the foods from the nourishing foods list. What are your observations from eating these nourishing foods?

LESSON 10
God Comforts Us

My journal often feels like a broken record. The same beautiful song is recorded in my journal over and over. Many of the "God moment" stories are about all the random and not-so-random times when I would read something in the Bible exactly when I needed to read it. God often seems to communicate to me, and maybe you, in this way. The story I am about to share is about one of those times when God spoke to me through a Bible verse. Please understand, I need to be a little vague with this story since I don't want to share anything too personal about someone else.

This "God moment" happened during a time when fear was overtaking my day, and I was experiencing immense fear in the pit of my stomach. It was so strong; it was almost painful. You see, I had to speak with someone about a conflict the following day. Have you ever had to have a difficult conversation where your words may seriously hurt someone if they are not chosen carefully? Did you feel scared about having to have the conversation? I know I sure did! We had to somehow resolve this conflict, and I wanted to resolve it with love. What if things were said that shouldn't be said? What if I got defensive and lashed out during the talk? I prayed for

God to give me strength to do and say the right things during this difficult conversation.

Then I Found Comfort in God

On this very same day, not once but twice, I stumbled upon lessons about trusting God when I'm afraid. The most impactful moment occurred when I was reading our nightly children's devotional, *God and Me*, to my son. On this particular day, the children's devotional pulled just two sentences out of the Bible (Mark 4:40). It simply said, "Why are you so afraid? Do you still have no faith?"

These words hit me smack in the heart and comforted my fearful soul. The fact that these two sentences were written in our devotional on the same day I was overwhelmed by fear made me feel like the words were being whispered to me, as if God were saying I could trust Him. God's got this!

When it was time to enter the room where the conversation was about to take place, I paused and prayed for God to guide my words and help me remain calm. Do you know what happened when I entered that room? A calm swept over me. I could feel the calmness move through my whole body. I felt protected. I just knew if any harsh words were said, the words were not going to hurt me. Somehow, God was shielding me from hurtful words. I was able to remain calm and compassionate the entire time. God was with us both during the whole conversation. Of course, the conflict wasn't resolved that day, but because I never said anything I would regret, we were able to resolve the conflict a few months later.

We all face hard conversations sometimes. This is an example of how praying before speaking helped me speak with love. Like all of us, I have had to have other difficult conversations at times, but the times when I didn't pray beforehand, I was not able to remain as calm and said things I now regret. This is why praying before everything is so important!

My Prayer

Thank you, God, for finding ways to speak to me and guide me. I don't know what I would do without your comfort and guidance. I am sorry for my lack of trust and for all the many times I fell short. Thank you for guiding me and loving me anyway. Amen.

Discussion Questions

1. Have you ever read a Bible verse that seemed to be exactly what you needed to hear? How did that make you feel?
2. What truth about God did you get from my story?
3. How do you relate to the Bible verse mentioned in my story? Are there times when you have trouble trusting God? What brings you comfort during those times?

Weekly Challenge

Read from the Bible every day this week. Any verses you want. Just read and think about how what you're reading is speaking to you.

Discuss Last Week's Challenge

Last week, you were challenged to encourage someone with your words. How did you carry out this challenge? How did it make you feel?

LESSON 11
God Speaks to Us

A group of my friends from church had been meeting up once a month for years to talk about one of my favorite subjects: books. Book club nights were sacred. We would talk for hours. Once, the last guest didn't leave until 1:00 a.m.! It was one of those special book club nights. The book club girls were all gathered in my kitchen, just catching up on all of our summer happenings. I was telling everyone about my son's latest ninja warriors camp adventures. "His favorite part is when he gets to run up the warped wall," I was saying when the doorbell rang.

Who Could That Be?
Must be someone new to the book club since this crowd usually doesn't bother to ring the doorbell … or knock, for that matter, I thought to myself as I opened the door.

A young man was standing on the front porch with a bag full of books slung over his shoulder and two books in his hand. "Hey," he said. As he spoke, he moved his arms forward to show the two books in his hands. "I am selling these books to raise money for my college tuition. We are asking for a twenty-dollar donation or more … or less … or whatever you want to give for the books."

I looked down at the books as he presented them. One of the books was written by an RD (registered dietitian), and the other one was a Christian book about having a peaceful mind. Out of all the books in his bag, he had chosen these two books to present to me. "I think God wants me to buy these books," I bluntly blurted out.

Pay very close attention here because this is the important part.

"You see," I began, "this isn't just any book club social we're having right now. This is a mindfulness and health book club social. I am a registered dietitian who writes a blog about health, faith, and mindfulness. One of books in your hands is about healthy foods written by a registered dietitian, and the other is a faith-based mindful peace book!"

He smiled but was calm and polite, showing little reaction to my amazed outburst. We talked a little more about where he went to school and the other books in his bag. I was intrigued by another book he had and asked him about it—I can't quite remember the name of it now. Although I wanted that book as well, I decided to stick with the first two. I paid him, and as he was leaving, I said, "I'm probably going to write a blog about this whole experience."

When I went back into the house, I told my friends about the awesome encounter. I showed them my books and told them about the one book I had wanted but didn't buy. We were all excited about the events that had just unfolded. We began the book club social filled with joy.

Two Hours Later ...

"Bye, thanks for coming!" I called out to my friends as they left my house.

I picked up the plates and was putting the plates in the sink when one of my friends came back into the house. "Lacy, you know that other book you had wanted?"

"Yes?" I replied.

"The guy selling the books left it on your front porch!" she exclaimed.

"What? That's amazing!" I felt like he had left that book as a way of saying he had, in fact, felt the significance of what transpired between us as well. I was truly amazed!

Thank God for Those Unexplainable Moments

That young man's kindness touched my heart. I went to bed so thankful for God and for those unexplainable little "God moments" in our lives.

The next morning, I awoke overcome with emotion. I fell on my knees, cried, and prayed, thanking God for the events of last night. I prayed for the young man, his school, and my book club friends. I hope I never forget the conversation the three of us had on that front porch. The young man and I physically talked, but God's quiet whisper was the loudest and most beautiful voice of all.

Soon after purchasing those books, I began reading the one written by the dietitian. Afterward, I was even more convinced I was meant to read this book!

I was a registered dietitian who had felt lead to combine my nutrition knowledge with my faith on a blog, "Mindfulness in Faith and Food." At the time of purchasing this book, I was in the process of writing my first faith-based nutrition book, and I was nervous about how it would go. On the first page of the dietitian's book—her acknowledgment page—she wrote about following her passion as God leads her and looking to God for guidance in every situation. Later in the book, she discussed the positive impact faith has on our health. When I bought this book, I knew I was buying a book by a registered dietitian, but I had no idea she talked about her faith in the book as well! Doesn't that make this story even more amazing?

Discussion Questions

1. Have you ever felt like God was speaking to you or guiding you? If so, in what way?
2. How would pausing before making a decision or entering a new place help you notice God's guidance?
3. 1 Kings 19:12 (NIV) says, "After the earthquake came a fire, but the Lord was not in the fire. And after the fire came a gentle whisper." What does this Bible verse say about how God sometimes might communicate with us?

Weekly Challenge

This week, try pausing and praying before making any big decisions.

Discuss Last Week's Challenge

Last week, you were challenged to read a Bible verse every day. Did anything you read stand out for you? If so, in what way?

LESSON 12
God Gives Us Opportunities

The Quick Prayer

"Class shouldn't be too long tonight," I said as I was leaving the house to teach nutrition to a group of college freshman. I figured I would be home shortly since this was the first class of the semester. I usually just go over the syllabus and class expectation on the first day.

As I was driving to work, I noticed a policeman carrying a gas canister to a car stopped on the side of the road. I thought to myself, Oh, that's nice. That driver must have run out of gas, and the policeman brought a canister of gas to the stranded driver.

This made my mind wonder, as it often does. I began to wonder how often I was too busy to notice others in need of some help or assistance. For some reason, I suddenly felt the need to pray a very specific prayer. "God, if I pass by someone on the side of the road who has run out of gas, please help me notice and help me do the right thing." Then I went to teach my students.

As predicted, my class was short. I was glad since I had lots to do at home. So I jumped in my car and headed home. On the way, I kid you not, I saw a car on the side of the road! A mother and her middle-school-aged son were standing beside the car. What was the likelihood I would pass by a car on the side of the road not long after saying that prayer?

I am going to tell you the truth about how I reacted at first, even though I am embarrassed. My first thought was, *Are you kidding me? Am I really supposed to stop now?*

But I had just prayed to God about that very thing that afternoon. I specifically asked God to help me notice others in need and help me do the right thing. Well, I noticed, and now I had to choose to do the right thing. So I pulled over and asked, "Are y'all okay? Do y'all need anything?"

The mother said, "We ran out of gas."

Is that not something! How often is someone stuck on the side of the road because they ran out of gas? Their car battery wasn't dead, and their car wasn't broken down for any other reason. I asked God to help me notice if someone ever runs out of gas, and here in front of me was this mother and son standing with a car with no gas!

Filling Their Tank and Filling My Heart

I responded, "Okay, hold on. I will get y'all some. I'll be right back."

Did God know these people were going to need gas at this time? Did God find a way to encourage me to stop for this family? I don't know. I don't even understand. I just know it happened, and I still remember the look of shocked appreciation on her son's face when I came back with a canister of gas. Their appreciation, and God's answer to my prayer filled my heart that day. As I filled the tank, my heart was filling up too.

We are all connected as children of God, so when we are kind to strangers, we are, in actuality, being kind to our brothers and sisters. What a gift to be able to help God's children, my family, and God's world in a small way! It is human nature to want to make an impact on the world and connect with others. When givers and receivers share an act of kindness with each other, a connection occurs. Humans have the ability to feel what others are feeling. This is called "empathy." So when we contribute to someone's happiness, we can actually experience the feelings they are feeling. Simply put, we can improve our own moods by showing kindness.

Your God Moments

I am so thankful God leads me because my decisions would be very different without Him. I believe that He is not a silent God. He wants to have a real relationship with us and wants to be a part of our lives. You don't have to say the perfect prayer for God to show up. He doesn't have to be manipulated to be in our lives because He wants to be in our lives! I have found this to be true in my own life. Many times, God has shown up!

God is compassionate. God loves us and doesn't have to be convinced to do something for us. Sometimes, all we need to do is ask, be patient, and mindfully watch. Get ready because God will show up!

Discussion Questions

1. What are some reasons we choose not to help someone? Read Luke 10:25–37 (NIV). Do you think the men who didn't stop may have chosen not to stop for similar reasons?
2. If we paused and prayed before going anywhere, would we be more helpful? Why or why not?
3. Do you think God gives us opportunities to spread love and kindness? Are we sometimes too busy to notice these opportunities? Would pausing and praying help us notice others in need more often?

Weekly Challenge

Help someone this week. It doesn't matter who; just help someone.

Discuss Last Week's Challenge

Did you have any big decisions to make last week? Did you find praying about the decision helpful?

LESSON 13
God Reassures Us

On January 27, 2017, my great aunt passed away. Aunt Kay had no children, and her husband was already waiting for her on the other side. Although she had no family of her own, she had loved all her nieces and nephews, and they had loved her, including my mom. In fact, my mom felt strongly that Aunt Kay would have wanted her to speak at the funeral. The catch was my mom did not like public speaking! I honestly couldn't believe my mom was really planning on saying something at the funeral. This was just so out of character for her. She even wrote several pages of beautiful words about Aunt Kay. Still, my mom said she had an exit plan if she got nervous. She said that if she walked up to the podium and realized she couldn't do it, she would just thank everyone for coming and then sit back down.

The day of the funeral was bright and beautiful, albeit windy. When I say windy, I mean windy! The wind never let up during the graveside funeral. The awnings were flapping, papers were rattling, and the wind was howling. I had trouble hearing the pastor or anything else. My mom later told me she had been so afraid the wind was going to distract her while she was trying to speak.

But then a miracle happened.

When the pastor called my mom to the podium, my mom stood up, and the wind abruptly stopped. It was instant! My mom spoke calmly and clearly and said everything she had planned to say, and the wind stayed silent the whole time. Once she was finished, the wind whooshed through the awnings, papers, and trees again, as if it were applauding.

I just sat there, amazed! What ... just ... happened? I thought. Even other people at the funeral had noticed and mentioned it to my mom.

What beautiful reassurance during a time we had to say a temporary "goodbye" to our loved one.

Discussion Questions

1. What is the significance of this story?
2. What truth about God is revealed in this story?
3. John 3:16 (NIV) says, "For God so loved the world that he gave his one and only Son, that whoever believes in him shall not perish but have eternal life." How does this Bible verse provide you comfort about life after death?

Weekly Challenge

Do you know of someone who has lost a loved one—or is just sad in general—and may need a little kindness? Send them a card just to say you are thinking of them this week.

Discuss Last Week's Challenge

Last week, you were challenged to help someone. Talk about the experience. How did it make you feel? Do you have any other ideas on how to help others in the future? Share your ideas.

LESSON 14
God Guides Us

One day, my children and I were close to being late to church. My husband, who is in the church band, was already at church. As we rushed into the lobby, I noticed a large table filled with at least thirty or forty pictures of adorable children from all over the world.

After church, I went to the table and learned that the children in the pictures were in need of financial help. Church members could choose to provide monthly financial help by sponsoring a child. Once you signed up to be a sponsor, you would send the child's family much needed money as well as notes and letters of encouragement. I was immediately drawn to a little boy named Matt from another country. I'm not exactly sure why I was drawn to him. He was definitely cute, but they all were cute. Perhaps it was something about his eyes. He was looking right into the camera as if he was looking right into my soul. I wanted to sponsor him, but I knew I needed to see if my husband would want to sponsor him as well. Perhaps he didn't even want to take on the responsibility of sponsoring a child. So I asked him if he wanted to go to the table and check it out. I didn't want to pressure him or even suggest a particular child to him. I just wanted to see what he thought without my interference.

When we walked over, my husband picked up only one picture and said, "What about this child?" The picture was of Matt! I couldn't believe it. We both chose Matt on our own. The choice was easy. We knew Matt was the child God wanted us to sponsor. To this day, we continue to sponsor and pray for Matt and his family.

Discussion Questions
1. Have you ever felt God guide you? In what way?
2. Has there ever been a time when you ignored God's guidance? If so, how did that choice affect you?
3. Galatians 5:25 (NLT) says, "Since we are living by the Spirit, let us follow the Spirit's leading in every part of our lives." What truth does this verse teach us about the Holy Spirit? How does this verse relate to this story?

Weekly Challenge
This week, specifically pray for God to guide you. Take notice of when you feel His guidance and remember to trust Him to lead you down the right path.

Discuss Last Week's Challenge
Did you get a chance to send a card to someone last week? Share the thoughts and feelings you had during this challenge.

LESSON 15
God Follows Through

In my experience, when God leads us to do something, He usually helps us get it done. I'm not saying hard times won't happen. I'm not saying we won't go through pain, but when God leads us to do something, He will be with us to make it happen.

There was a time when our church was trying to pay off a debt for the new children's building. The building provided a larger place for our growing groups of children. Once it was built, our church wanted to reduce the debt and free up the church finances so we could serve our community and God's world in other ways. My husband and I wanted to contribute. In fact, we felt that, as members of the church, it was our duty to help pay the bills just as it was our duty to pay the mortgage of our home. We just were not sure of the amount we should contribute.

When we had bought our own home, we had cut back on some things because we wanted that home. Our home was more important than most of the stuff we had cut out of our lifestyle. We felt the same about our church home.

My husband and I prayed and hoped that God would lead us. Afterward, we finally came up with an amount that seemed hard for us, but we wanted to practice putting God before our own material desires. We had just bought a home, and we had planned on renovating the living room, but we were now going to postpone the renovations for three years in order to give to our church.

We didn't do this in order to get something in return, but something exciting did happen.

Follow God without Expectations

Before I go on, I want to explain what I am not saying. I am not saying that every time you sacrifice, God rewards you with money. Many times, people have sacrificed for God, even their lives, and didn't receive money as a result. But sometimes, I think God does show us just how much we can trust Him to take care of us.

When we trust God, He finds a way to show us His presence. When God leads us to do His will, He helps us get it done.

We Followed and God Helped Us Get It Done

My husband and I made a pledge that would not leave us struggling but rather would make us have to hold off on some spending. After we took that leap of faith and pledged our financial giving to the church, my husband received an unexpected raise at work and found out that he was getting some backpay money he didn't know he had coming!

Giving Changed Our Priorities

You know what was funny? During the process of giving to the church, we realized we didn't need the elaborate renovation we had originally planned. We were happy. We had a perfectly functioning kitchen. We had a cozy, climate-controlled house, and we had laughter and love filling all the rooms. Fancy renovations would change the things about life that actually made us the happiest. With this unexpected money, we were able to do a less elaborate renovation in two years instead of three and could give an extra financial gift to our church as a Christmas gift.

Honestly, I had to bite my tongue when my husband said, "Yeah, I think I am going to give this extra money to the church." I wanted to say, But when it is time to pay that last chunk of money we pledged to the church, aren't you going to wish you had kept this money? But I knew this was something good my husband wanted to do, so I held back from saying anything.

But Wait, It Gets Even Better!

So we gave that extra money without counting it toward the pledge. But a few months later, our pledge was due, and—just as I had predicted—we were kicking ourselves for not counting the Christmas gift as part of our pledge. You would think we would have been better at trusting God after all this, but when it was time for our last payment to the campaign, we were extremely nervous! It was year three of the campaign, and we had one big chunk of our pledge to give. Oh, did I mention that the amount we had given at Christmas was the amount we had left to give?

So, with heavy hearts, we reluctantly wrote a check and gave the last sum to the church.

No, Really, It Does Get Better ... Bring On the Arm Chills!

You know what happened the very next week? My husband was asked to do an extra, one-time, big job at work that paid him almost the exact amount we had given to the church! I mean, wow ... just wow! We didn't get loads and loads of extra money, but we got the money we needed to serve God and our brothers and sisters at our church.

One day, I hope to have more trust in God because He keeps blowing me away. All I can say is God follows through!

Discussion Questions

1. In what ways could you let go and trust God more in your life?
2. How would trusting God more relieve stress and anxiety?
3. Psalms 46:10 (ESV) says, "Be still, and know that I am God. I will be exalted among the nations, I will be exalted in the earth!" Romans 8:28 (ESV) says, "And we know that for those who love God all things work together for good, for those who are called according to his purpose." And Joshua 1:9 (ESV) says, "Have I not commanded you? Be strong and courageous. Do not be frightened, and do not be dismayed, for the Lord your God is with you wherever you go." These Bible verses are about trusting God. In your own words, what does each Bible verse say about trusting God?

Weekly Challenge

In a journal, write down something that is worrying you. Next, write each Bible verse listed above and relate the verses to your worry. Then pray to God for help and guidance.

Discuss Last Week's Challenge

Last week, you were challenged to ask God to guide you. Did you notice God's guidance? In what way?

LESSON 16
God Amazes Us

I don't even know exactly how to explain what happened, so I am just going to tell this story and let you decide how to interpret.

The Miscarriage ... Then My Son Was Born

In 2009, my beautiful little boy was born. Just over a year earlier, I'd had a miscarriage. My body had held on to my first baby for three months. I still have my only picture via an ultrasound of my first baby, and I can still remember seeing the little heartbeat on the ultrasound. I will always love that first baby, and as you can imagine, I was over the moon to find out I was pregnant again so soon after. I worried for just a few days about a miscarriage happening, but just like that time many years ago in middle school, I experienced this unspoken whisper from God. I felt like God was telling me this baby was going to be born. Again, like in middle school, I had this feeling of elated joy!

Thankfully, the delivery of my son went well. He was a healthy baby except for a minor hydrocele. The doctors said this was not unusual and that the hydrocele usually goes away before the age of one. However, if the hydrocele did not go away by the time my son was a year old, then he may need minor surgery, especially if the hydrocele turned into a hernia.

What in the World Was Happening?

A year went by, and before we knew it, we were celebrating my little boy's first birthday. Soon after, I noticed a little redness when I was changing my son's diaper. Knowing about the hydrocele, I decided to get him checked out. We took him to the doctor, and to my surprise, the doctor recommended we go straight to the urologist. It was now after 5:00 p.m., and the doctor was going to meet us at his already closed office. I started thinking the worst.

On the way to the urologist, my son suddenly projectile vomited all over the car, car seat, and me. What in world was happening?

The urologist concluded that my son did have a hernia and needed surgery, but thankfully, this was not an emergency. The surgery could be scheduled for a later date. During the procedure, my son would be put to sleep for a couple of hours, and then he would go home the same day of the surgery.

Whew, crisis averted ... but as the days for the surgery drew nearer, I began to worry again. My logical mind knew this was a minor surgery, but the protective mother in me began to panic as the day approached. I had heard of babies having bad reactions to anesthesia, and by the night before the surgery, I was extremely stressed, although, I still did my normal bedtime routine just as I always did. First, I lay my son on the changing table to change his diaper and put on his pajamas. Then I bowed my head and said a prayer while he was still lying on the changing table. This time, I said a special prayer, asking God to please help us know He was there with us and would be right there with us during the surgery. I really, really needed reassurance that God was with us.

Afterward, I picked up my son and carried him to the rocking chair so we could read our bedtime stories. He was looking at me and smiling as we went to the chair. Then his gaze shifted to the ceiling, and he suddenly said, "Hey," as though he were greeting someone.

I was puzzled and curiously asked, "Who are you talking to?"

My one-year-old son simply replied, "God."

Bring On Those Chills

Chills ran up my arm. My mouth dropped open. I could barely move or focus on the book I was reading to my son. In awe, I asked myself, What ... just ... happened? My son was not even two years old yet. How did he know God was with him all the time?

I don't know how my son knew God was there, and I am not sure how he knew he could just say "hey" to God anytime. I just know that I prayed for God to help us know He was there, and He did!

The surgery went smoothly, and my son was home in a few hours, healthy once more.

Discussion Questions

1. Do you think God still speaks to us today? Have you ever felt God speaking to you? In what ways has God found a way to speak to you?

2. Have you ever felt completely in awe after witnessing something God had done? What did you learn from that experience?

3. Matthew 19:26 (ESV) says that "with God all things are possible." What does this Bible verse say about God and miracles?

Weekly Challenge

Take the time to talk to God this week. Find a quiet place and simply pray and listen for at least ten minutes each day.

Discuss Last Week's Challenge

Last week, you were asked to write about something you are worrying about, then pray for God's help and guidance. How are you emotionally dealing with this worry right now? Were you able to give your worry to God, or do you still struggle? Either answer is okay. God will never leave you regardless.

LESSON 17
God Knows

$\mathcal{I}$ couldn't believe what was happening. I was following an ambulance that was carrying my kindergartener to the hospital. My then six-year-old son, Hilt, was taking this ambulance ride from urgent care to the hospital. Before that ride, he had been on antibiotics but just kept getting sicker.

When we arrived at the ER, the doctors diagnosed him with pneumonia and admitted him to the hospital. While in the hospital, they tested him for viruses to see what could have caused the pneumonia. They found that he had two different strains of the common cold viruses. That was it. Nothing fancy, just the little old common cold was causing all this drama. He stayed in the hospital battling the pneumonia for five days. Finally, everything seemed cleared up, and he was ready to be released to go home.

The next six months were a whirlwind. After being released, his cough just kept coming back. A few days after getting the cough again, he would get a fever. This was happening about every two to three weeks.

Knowing this wasn't normal, the doctors scheduled an X-ray. The X-ray showed that he had a collapsed lung, which had developed from all these lung issues. It was now June, six months after being released from the hospital for pneumonia, and my son was still coughing, struggling to breathe when he ran, getting tired easily, and getting frequent fevers. He had taken so many antibiotics that I had lost count. He had been put to sleep twice for minor lung procedures.

The doctors decided to get a CT scan to see if he had a condition called bronchiectasis, which is defined as abnormal widening of the bronchi or their branches, causing a risk of infection.[45] The damage to the lungs is considered permanent. The CT scan confirmed he did indeed have this condition.

I had never heard of it, so, of course, I looked it up online. The things I read terrified me. I read about people needing to permanently carry an oxygen tank around at a young age and that the frequency of infection can damage the lungs even more over time. I also read that the life expectancy could be shorter if the bronchiectasis started when someone was a child and was severe. Fortunately, as I discovered later, many of these worst-case scenarios were for people whose bronchiectasis was caused by another ongoing chronic condition, not by one strange incident like in Hilt's case. In fact, Hilt's case was unusual. It was so unusual that Hilt became a case study for medical students in Chapel Hill.

I was not handling the diagnosis well. I walked around constantly on the verge of crying but trying to seem cheerful for my children. Many nights, I prayed and let out all my pent-up tears. I feared what this meant for my son. I can't even bring myself to type all the worries I was feeling, but if you are a parent, you can probably imagine the fears that went through my head during this time.

I Wanted to Cancel

The very same week I learned of the diagnosis, I wanted to shut myself off from everyone, but our church book club was supposed to meet at my house! I came inches from canceling. Most of the book club regulars were not able to come, so I started thinking no one was going to show up anyway. But then a new girl sent me an email saying she would like to come and bring two of her friends. I couldn't cancel when new people had expressed interest, so I decided to just push through. The funny thing was the new girl, who had originally expressed interest, was unable to attend due to a prior commitment, but her two friends did come.

These two girls, who only attended this one time, probably didn't know what they were walking into. I was unorganized and monopolized the whole conversation. I ended up pouring all my emotions out to these brand-new people. They were such patient listeners, and although I don't know if they got much out of the book club, I felt much better after that night.

God's Perfect Timing

The doctors were trying all kinds of treatments. My son was now on continuous antibiotics three times a week and doing thirty-minute treatments twice a day. He had several procedures and X-rays during this time as well. But God, like so many times before, found a way to comfort us before the first of these procedures.

For this particular procedure, my son was going to the Levine's Children's Hospital where he would be put to sleep. The night before the procedure, my six-year-old asked, "Can we read some stories before I go to sleep?"

"Of course, let's read the *God and Me* book first," I replied as I snuggled with my little boy. I could tell my son was a little nervous as we opened the *God and Me* children's daily devotional to the page where we had left off. He was quiet and more clingy than usual. His voice was pleading, as if he were desperate for comfort.

Amazingly, the devotional for that night was about going to the hospital! It said, "Dear God, I'm thankful that You are always with me, even at the doctor's office or the hospital. Amen."

Even my son noticed the significance and couldn't believe that out of all the devotionals in the book, the one for that night talked about the hospital. In amazement my son exclaimed, "How does God do that?"

Smiling through tears, I replied, "I don't know how God does things like this, but I am sure glad God does!"

God's perfect timing indeed!

The procedure went well. Before I knew it, a year had gone by since receiving that initial diagnosis and pouring my heart out to those random new girls at the book club.

Can I Ask You a Weird Question?

The doctors decided it was time to talk about doing a surgery to remove the damaged lobe of my son's lung. This surgery was invasive but would hopefully cure my son of his bronchiectasis. The doctor gave us a list of surgeons, so I began to go down the list and making calls. I called the first office on the list to set up a consultation with a surgeon in Charlotte, North Carolina.

The receptionist started asking basic questions like, "What is the appointment for?" and "What is your home address?" Then she paused and said, "Can I ask you a weird question?"

I thought, This is an unusual question from a receptionist. What in the world is she going to ask me? But all I said was, "Okay."

She said, "Do you happen to have a book club with St. John's in Rock Hill, South Carolina?"

Shocked and confused, I replied, "Yes!"

She then exclaimed, "I think I have been to your house!"

When I had been answering her questions over the phone, she remembered hearing a similar story a year earlier at a book club she had attended once. She then recognized the address I had just given her and figured out she and her friend—you know, that other new girl—who also worked in the same office, had been to my house the week my son had been diagnosed a year ago!

Knowing that people at the surgeon's office knew our story and family was such a comfort to me.

God's Plan to Bring Comfort and Guidance
Was Put into Action a Year Earlier!

After the phone call ended, I thought to myself, *Wow, the week my son was diagnosed a year ago, I was walking around terrified and wishing I would feel God's presence, but He was right there all along.*

I felt like God was giving me comfort during that book club night. Little did I know that same book club social would give me comfort a year later. Did God somehow help me cross paths with these ladies right when my son was diagnosed? Did He know this journey would lead to a big surgery way back then? Of *course* He did! Many of us have learned that God knows all, our past and our future, but to truly witness this was humbling.

This experience made me feel like God was giving me a warm hug. I could feel His presence and realized just how present He had been the whole time. As I processed this, the tears began running down my face and chills ran up my arm. Oh, and I didn't call any other surgeons on the list. We had found our surgeon as far as I was concerned.

Discussion Questions

1. In what ways did God provide comfort to me in this story?
2. What is the significance of something coming full circle a year later in this story? What does this story tell us about God?
3. Psalm 147:5 (ESV) says, "Great is our Lord, and abundant in power; his understanding is beyond measure." What does this Bible verse say about God's power and ability to know how something will affect your future?

Weekly Challenge

This story talks about how my friends and strangers listened while I monopolized the conversation. They were a blessing to me just by listening. This week, I challenge you to focus on listening to others. Focus on them, their feelings, and their interest while in conversation. Ask questions about them and be the listener.

Discuss Last Week's Challenge

Discuss your observations from your quiet prayer time last week. How did your conversation with God go? Did you take the time to listen as well as speak to Him?

LESSON 18
God Answers Us

My son had his surgery in August 2017. September was wonderful. He played soccer like he had never had bronchiectasis. Then in October, he developed a completely unrelated disease called HSP, or Henoch-Schonlein purpura, which is a disease involving inflammation of small blood vessels. As explained to me by Hilt's doctor, the inflammation causes blood vessels in the skin, intestines, kidneys, and joints to start leaking! My son's hands and feet swelled, and they hurt so badly that he needed to ride in a wheelchair to get to the doctor's office. He also had bruises all over his feet and legs, and he had to get his kidneys checked regularly.

The scariest thing for me was that this disease could last for as little as eight weeks to as long as several years and could potentially cause permanent damage to his organs. I just felt like I couldn't take another several years of battling yet another condition. My son had just gotten through a two-and-a-half-year battle with one disease; now he had to go through another? *Why is this happening again?* I thought over and over.

What Am I Doing Wrong?

It felt like God was mad at us for trying to get rid of one problem, so He gave my son another disease. As if He was saying, "Well, if you take the bronchiectasis away, then I will just give your son something else."

I kept thinking, *What am I doing wrong? Why is God punishing us?* You would think that I would have had more faith and trust after all the other times I had experienced the wonder of God's presence ... but I didn't. I was so terrified again. Yet, even as I lacked trust in God, He never abandoned me.

I was eating breakfast one day, and an awful thought swiftly and briefly passed through my head. It was the opposite of "I love you, God." I can't even bring myself to write the words.

As soon as those words ran through in my head, I immediately panicked and said aloud, "I didn't mean that! I am so sorry, God. I *do* love you." And I was telling the truth. I did truly love God. In fact, I loved Him so much that it hurt. In truth, I would not have been so upset with God if I didn't love Him so much. You know how we get more upset when we feel like the ones we love have abandoned us? That was what I had been feeling. I don't feel nearly as hurt when a stranger does something I dislike, but when a loved one disappoints me ... it's painful.

Honestly, those hateful thoughts scared me. I started thinking, *I really don't want to make God cross with me, so I better make sure I am saying pleasing things. I mean, look at all the pain I'm already going through! What more is God going to do to me now that I had this awful thought?* Although I will never stop feeling guilty for thinking those words, I know that, in reality, I was quite literally a child lashing out at a parent.

If you are a parent, you have probably heard at least one of your children say, "I hate you!" when you don't do what they want. I know I have heard it a couple of times. When my kids have yelled these words at me, I always knew they loved me and were really saying, "I am angry and in pain."

Surprisingly, I still hadn't hit rock bottom yet. I was angry, but I still had faith and hope. I continued to pray for God's help. It wasn't until a few days later that I felt like I was finally losing my ability to cope and function.

The Desperate Prayer

On that night, I prayed one of the most desperate prayers I had ever prayed. My children had just fallen asleep, so I crept into the hallway near them and prayed with great desperation and fear. I told God how I was feeling, and I cried, telling God that the pain and stress were just too much. I was worried not only about my son's physical health, but also his emotional health. My son, who had handled the first condition with resilience, had started randomly saying the last few days, "I feel sad, and I don't know why." Well, I knew why. Being sick again was taking its toll on him.

During this desperate prayer, I talked to God about all this. I was raw and honest with Him about how I was feeling. After I prayed this foxhole prayer, I went into my son's room and prayed over him while he slept.

Then I cried myself to sleep.

God Can Find Ways to Speak to Us

The next morning, my son's bruises looked even worse! It was yet another Sunday we wouldn't make it to church. We hadn't been to church in a month because of this painful disease.

That night, I was a wreck. I was both angry and felt this shift in my faith and not in a good way. Feeling hopeless, I texted my friend Lollie. I told her I didn't think asking God for help did anything, so I was going to quit asking. Lollie, who happened to be our pastor's wife, let me vent. She didn't try to convince to feel differently. She mostly listened and expressed understanding for why I felt the way

I did. How great it is to have a friend who accepts you even at your worst! I knew I still loved God as a child does when they're mad at their parent, but I didn't think He was going to help me. Although I had given up on God for help, He had not given up on me.

Here is the thing. Sure, I had pleaded to God to listen and answer me, but at the same time, I didn't make it easy for God to speak to me. Remember, I hadn't been to church in a month due to this disease. I also finished my devotional about two months earlier and hadn't picked out another one yet. In the past, when I was going through something, a sermon, devotional, or Bible verse seemed to somehow speak about exactly what I was going through. In other words, when I was actively seeking God, He always seemed to communicate with me. But I currently wasn't reading or listening to anything about God ... until that Tuesday.

A while back, I had purchased some Christian conversation starter cards as a Christmas present for my children. On Tuesday, these cards came in the mail. My son was stuck in bed, so I decided to give this Christmas present a little early. We opened the present that Tuesday night and decided to try one of them right away.

The first card we grabbed said, "Have you ever prayed a foxhole prayer like the one Jonah prayed in Jonah 2:1?"

Although I had heard the term before, I decided to look up the actual definition of foxhole. A foxhole is "a pit dug usually hastily for individual cover from enemy fire."[46] After reading this and other descriptions, I gathered that a foxhole prayer is one you pray in utter desperation and fear like soldiers have prayed in the foxhole during war.[47] I was speechless! I had just prayed a foxhole prayer, and I was currently struggling with the results of it. Because I felt like God was not answering my foxhole prayer, my doubts and fears were overwhelming me!

I wondered what the foxhole prayer was in Jonah 2:1. I frantically it looked up, and it read, "From inside the fish Jonah prayed to the Lord his God. He said: 'In my distress I called to the Lord, and He answered me. From deep in the realm of the dead I called for help, and You listened to my cry'" (NIV).

I can barely describe what I was feeling when I read those words. I guess the best way to describe it is utter relief.

Let Me Just Recap for a Moment

I prayed a foxhole prayer and "in my distress, I called to the Lord." By Sunday night, I had decided God wouldn't answer me. Then, the very next Bible verse I randomly read was about how God listened and answered Jonah's distressed "foxhole prayer"! I was humbled, ashamed, relieved, and encouraged all at once. I had doubted that God would answer my foxhole prayer, and then I felt like He said, "I am answering your foxhole prayer."

God shows me over and over and over that He is listening and answering, but I am still so quick to doubt over and over and over. You know what amazes me the most? God stays by my side even when I don't deserve it, and He continues to show me love and devotion. He continues to guide me and comfort me no matter how many times I fail to trust Him. What a comfort to know that whether I say the right or wrong things, God still loves and leads me. Whether I trust or doubt, God is still comforting me, just as a parent does for their child. Even when our children mess up, we continue to love, comfort, and help them. Looks like God really does do the same for us!

When my son was first diagnosed with HSP, I tried to pray the "right" things to make God love me, listen to me, and help me. Turns out, even when I said the wrong things, I couldn't make God stop loving me, listening to me, or helping me. What a relief that was! Although I will continue to try to do what God wants, I know I will continue to fail over and over and over. I will be selfish, lack trust, and be quick to anger sometimes. And I won't always praise God in the storm, but, regardless, He is constant.

Fortunately, my son did go into remission and has been in remission for over two years now. Many times, HSP doesn't come back.

Discussion Questions

1. What does this story tell us about God's love and forgiveness?
2. Do you think God answers every prayer? Explain your answer.
3. Romans 5:8 (NIV) says, "But God demonstrates his own love for us in this: While we were still sinners, Christ died for us." What does this verse say about God's love for us even when we mess up?

So Where Are We Now?

My children are doing great. My daughter is busy with dance competitions, and my son is loving life on a travel soccer team.

As for me, I am still learning and growing every day. I'm still trying to live a life that glorifies God and supports others while having a little fun in the process. I am still messing up regularly, but faith-based mindfulness and nutrition has certainly helped me more than anything else I have found to get back on track with my health and faith. Now I am in the best shape of my life, enjoying my food, and fueling my brain and body so I can have as much strength as possible to serve God and others. How amazingly freeing that is! I get to eat without feeling deprived, eat delicious foods I love, and feed my mind, body, and soul with healing nutrient-dense foods, and I feel so good! But most importantly, by incorporating mindfulness into my diet and life, I am able to notice God all around me a little more often. I am finally beginning to understand in my heart what I knew in my head. Health is about more than weight. Health is about feeding our mind, body, *and* soul.

Your Challenge as You Go Forward

Now that this study has come to an end, I give you a new challenge: to glorify God in all that you do. Wherever you are and whatever you are doing, whether eating or just living your daily life, take time to enjoy it all. Pause and notice the presence of God. Pray before entering any new place, and when you pray, remember to notice the good things God has given you and be thankful. Ask for guidance and for God to help you show love to whomever you meet. Each day, take the time to have quiet time with God. Read the Bible and write in a journal. When you eat, mindfully choose foods that will nourish the body God created and then take the time to enjoy eating God's gift in His presence.

When it comes to journaling, I recommend trying the accompanying *Transforming the Mind, Body, & Soul*. This 30-day journal was designed to help you put the practices in this book into action in your daily life. The prompts in the journal are the very components I recommend including in your own journal as you work to transform your health through faith-based mindfulness and nutrition. This enjoyable, relaxing, and uplifting journal guides your writing, so you are thinking about all the components of this faith-based mindfulness and nutrition approach to life.

Go enjoy life and stay healthy in every way possible!

APPENDIX A

$\mathcal{B}$eing adequately nourished and feeling your best is going to help with fatigue and energy; therefore, everything included will help improve energy and feelings of fatigue.

List of Nutrients and Their Benefits

Antioxidants

- Reduce oxidative stress and protect your cells from free radicals[48]
- Promote gut health[49]
- Promote a healthy immune system[50]
- Have anti-inflammatory properties[51]
- Help with mood disorders, like depression, anxiety, and stress[52]
- Have cancer-fighting properties[53]
- Reduce risk of heart disease and stroke[54]
- Promote healthy skin and hair[55]
- May reduce cognitive decline and the risk of Alzheimer's and dementia[56]
- Aid in addiction recovery[57]

- May help with symptoms of ADHD and autism—more research is needed[58]
- May help with asthma and seasonal allergies[59]
- Reduce risk of developing degenerative and autoimmune diseases[60]
- May reduce joint pain and arthritis[61]

Examples of antioxidants include the following: vitamin A, vitamin E, vitamin C, polyphenols, flavonoid polyphenols, selenium, glutathione, quercetin, and kaempferol (flavonoids), sulforaphane, EGCG—found in green tea—and anthocyanins.

While all antioxidants provide the above benefits, each antioxidant has its own strengths. For example, sulforaphane and anthocyanins appear particularly beneficial when it comes to cancer prevention.[62] The phytochemicals in apples are linked to better asthma and seasonal allergy control.[63]

Antioxidant-rich anti-inflammatory foods include:
- Fruits and vegetables, especially berries and dark leafy greens
- Beans
- Nuts and seeds, including nut and seed butter
- Nutritional yeast
- Herbs and spices like thyme, turmeric, rosemary, cinnamon, ginger, sage, garlic, and cilantro[64]
- Dark chocolate
- Black tea, green tea, matcha tea, chamomile tea, and olive leaf tea
- Extra virgin olive oil
  - Note: different oils have different positive characteristics. Olive oil, almond oil, and avocado oil are a great source of monounsaturated fats. Coconut oil is a good source of MCT (medium-chain triglycerides)

oil. Research suggests that MCT oils are metabolized differently and are not stored as fat. MCT oil may even slightly increase metabolism[65].

Some oils have a beneficial omega-3 and omega-6 ratio. Omega-3 and omega-6 are important for the body. However, the ratio between these two polyunsaturated fats is also very important. Here in the United States, we are getting more omega-6 compared to omega-3. In other words, we are getting too much omega-6 and not enough omega-3s. We should aim for at max a four to one omega-6 to omega-3 ratio. In the US, the ratio is anywhere from twelve to one to twenty-five to one! These high omega-6 ratios promote inflammation.[66] Flax seed oil has a one to four omega-6 to omega-3 ratio!

B Vitamins

Such vitamins include B1 (thiamine), B2 (riboflavin), B3 (niacin), B5 (pantothenic acid), B6, B7 (biotin), B12, and folic acid/folate.

Varying benefits of B vitamins include:

- Help with mood disorders, like depression, anxiety, and stress[67]
- Improved energy levels and fatigue[68]
- A healthy immune system[69]
- Improved GI Inflammation[70]
- Aid in addiction recovery[71]
- Healthy bones, muscles, and nerves[72]
  - o Note: deficiencies in vitamin B6, B12, and folic acid have been linked to increased symptoms of autism and ADHD.[73]

B vitamin-rich foods include:
- Salmon
- Chicken
- Turkey
- Free-range eggs
- Legumes
- Yogurt
- Nutritional yeast
- Dark leafy greens
- Whole grains
- Zucchini, squash, and avocado

Minerals

Potassium
- Potassium is needed for heart and muscle function and bone maintenance.
- It also helps maintain water and electrolyte balance in your body.
- Potassium deficiency can increase the risk of kidney stones, high blood pressure, and urinary calcium excretion.
- We usually get plenty in our diet; thus, potassium deficiency is rare.[74]

Potassium-rich foods include:
- White beans
- Potatoes
- Beets
- Yellow squash
- Bananas
- Spinach

Zinc

- Deficiency may increase depression, anxiety, and ADHD symptoms.[75]
- An adequate supply of zinc promotes a healthy immune system.[76]
- Zinc also aids in addiction recovery.[77]

Sources of zinc include:
- Oysters
- Crab
- Turkey
- Chicken
- Legumes and beans
- Cashews
- Sunflower seeds
- Broccoli
- Dark chocolate
- Quinoa
- Buckwheat
- Oats

Iron

- Iron promotes healthy immune function.[78]
- Deficiency causes anemia and fatigue and reduces the ability to fight off infections.[79]

Sources of iron include:
- Fish and shellfish
- Turkey
- Legumes
- Spinach, turnip greens, and collard greens
- Quinoa

Magnesium

- Magnesium supports healthy bones, muscles, and nerves.[80]
- Deficiencies are associated with increased anxiety symptoms, breast cancer, increased risk of heart disease and diabetes, lower lung function, and increased inflammation.[81]
- People with migraine headaches often have low magnesium levels.[82]

Magnesium-rich foods include:
- Salmon
- Whole grains
- Dark leafy greens
- Corn
- Dark chocolate
- Avocados
- Legumes, nuts, and seeds

Calcium

- Calcium is important for bone health.[83]

Calcium sources include:
- Dairy products
- Spinach
- Buckwheat

Fiber

Some fiber is prebiotic.[84] Good bacteria in the gut feeds on prebiotics; all prebiotics are fiber, but not all fiber is prebiotic Fiber also:.
- Reduces the risk of cancer.[85]
- Has anti-inflammatory properties.[86]
- Promotes healthy digestion.[87]
- Immune supportive[88].

- May reduce joint pain and arthritis inflammation.[89]
- Reduces the risk of heart disease and stroke.[90]
- Helps you feel full after eating; thus, helps with satiety and weight loss.[91]
- Helps with mood and mood disorders, like depression, anxiety, and stress.[92]
- Protects against diabetes.[93]

Fiber-rich foods include:
- Fruits and vegetables
- Whole grains
- Beans, nuts, and seeds

Other Fat-Soluble Vitamins

Vitamin D

Low levels of vitamin D have been associated with autoimmune diseases, skin issues, reduced immune function, poor gut health increased inflammation, decreased cognitive function in the elderly, cancer, mood disorders—like depression, anxiety, and stress—increased symptoms from ADD and ADHD, asthma and seasonal allergies, autism, joint pain, and arthritis.[94]

Sources of vitamin D include:
- Mushrooms that have been exposed to UV light
- Salmon
- Fortified milk

Vitamin K

- Vitamin K is important for bone health, heart disease, and blood clotting.[95]

Sources of vitamin K include:
- Dark leafy greens
- Avocados
- Broccoli
- Cabbage
- Asparagus
- Brussels sprouts
- Carrots
    - Note: if you are taking a blood thinner, you may have to decrease your vitamin K intake.

Healthy Fats

Omega-3 Polyunsaturated Fats
- May help with joint pain and arthritis.[96]
- Have anti-inflammatory properties.[97]
- Help with mood and mood disorders, like depression, anxiety, and stress.[98]
- Reduce the risk of heart disease.[99]
- Promote gut health.[100]
- May reduce cognitive decline and the risk of Alzheimer's and Dementia.[101]
- May improve memory.[102]
- Aid in addiction recovery.[103]
- May help with asthma and seasonal allergies.[104]
- May help with symptoms of ADHD and autism—more research is needed.[105]

Sources of DHA and EPA omega-3 are:
- Fatty fish like salmon and tuna
- Cage-free eggs

Sources of plant-based ALA omega-3s are:
- Extra virgin olive oil
- Kale
- Flaxseed
- Chia seed
- Spinach
- Walnuts and brussels sprouts
- Hemp seeds

Monounsaturated Fats
- Reduce the risk of heart disease.
- Promote a healthy immune system.
- May reduce cognitive decline and the risk of Alzheimer's and dementia.[106]

Sources of monounsaturated fats include:
- Tuna and salmon
- Avocado
- Walnuts, pistachios, almonds, flaxseed, sunflower seeds, and hemp seeds

Probiotics
- Promote gut health.[107]
- Support the immune system.[108]
- Have anti-inflammatory properties.[109]
- Help with mood and mood disorders like depression, anxiety, and stress.[110]
- Reduce the risk of cancer.[111]
- Reduce risk of heart disease and stroke.[112]
- May reduce cognitive decline and the risk of Alzheimer's and dementia.[113]
- May reduce the risk of some autoimmune diseases.[114]
- Aid in addiction recovery.[115]

- May help with asthma and seasonal allergies.[116]
- May improve ADHD symptoms and reduce risk of development with early intervention in newborns, although more research is needed.[117]

- Probiotic foods include:
- Sauerkraut
- Kimchi
- Fermented pickles
- Miso
- Kefir
- Tempeh
- Kombucha
- Greek yogurt

Prebiotics

Since prebiotics feed probiotics, they can indirectly have the same benefits as probiotics.

Prebiotics include:
- Mangoes
- Apples
- Tart cherries
- Blueberries
- Bananas
- Broccoli
- Cauliflower
- Turnip greens and collard greens
- Asparagus
- Carrots
- Brussels sprouts
- Oats
- Black beans

- Cannellini beans
- Green peas
- Chickpeas
- Flaxseed

L-theanine

- Anti-anxiety properties—relaxes or calms the brain without making you drowsy.[118]
- May improve mental focus and cognitive performance.[119]
- Supports the immune system.[120]

L-theanine sources are:
- Green tea and black tea

Beta Glucan

- Supports the immune system.[121]
- May help with asthma and seasonal allergies, according to preliminary studies.[122]

A beta glucan source is:
- Nutritional yeast

Melatonin—or Melatonin Precursors
Such as Tryptophan and Serotonin

- Promotes better sleep at night and relaxation during the day.[123]
- Aids in addiction recovery by promoting sleep.
  - Lack of sleep is linked to an increased risk of mood disorders and chronic diseases and conditions and decreased immune function as well as cognitive function.[124]

A melatonin source is:
- Tart cherries
    - o **Note:** according to research, tryptophan may not help with mood on its own, but it may be able to boost serotonin—a happy hormone—levels and thus mood when paired with a carbohydrate-rich food.[125] For tryptophan to work, this amino acid must first be absorbed. Unfortunately, tryptophan must compete with other amino acids to be absorbed. Carbohydrates promote amino acid absorption. Therefore, it may improve the absorption of tryptophan.

Sources of tryptophan include:
- Eggs
- Cheese
- Soy
- Salmon
- Nuts and seeds.
    - o **Note:** salmon and cage-free eggs are also good sources of omega-3 and vitamin D. Nuts are a good source of fiber and antioxidants as well.
- Chamomile tea
    - o According to research, chamomile tea improves sleep quality and reduces depression in sleep-disturbed individuals, especially postnatal women, and may help with generalized anxiety disorder. [126]

Foods That Can Have a Negative Impact on How We Feel, Think, and Function

These foods—refined sugar and refined carbohydrates, fried foods, alcohol, beer, butter, margarine, trans fat, vegetable oils, red meats, smoked meats, milk chocolate, and ultra-processed foods—promote the growth of "bad" bacteria in the gut and are inflammatory. Therefore, refined sugar may increase the risk for chronic conditions, including heart disease, strokes, Alzheimer's, dementia, and other brain dysfunctions; decrease immunity; increase inflammation and mood disorders, like depression, anxiety, and stress; exacerbate symptoms of ADHD and autism; hinder addiction recovery; increase the risk of cancer; and reduce brain function.[127]

Ultra-processed Foods

Limiting processed foods promotes gut balance; reduces the risk of Alzheimer's, dementia, cancer, and inflammation; and improves symptoms of ADHD. Heavily processed, low-fiber foods may reduce brain and immune function and contribute to depression, stress, and mood swings. [128]

However, not all "processed" foods are bad. Processing simply means altering a food. Pre-cut vegetables are considered processed because they were cut up, i.e., altered. However, heavily processed foods are the foods you want to limit. When reading the labels on food boxes, look for short ingredients lists with simple food listed. Look for whole foods like whole grains, vegetables, nuts, or fruit as the first ingredient on carbohydrate or starchy foods like crackers. Look for foods that have no added sugar or trans-fat. Heavily processed foods include pastries, sausage, salami, bologna, hot dogs, fruit snacks, candy, and some cereals.

Food Sensitivities and Intolerances

Food sensitivities and intolerances can contribute to poor gut health, and inversely, poor gut health can increase food sensitivities.[129] Changing your diet can greatly improve your gut health and many symptoms and conditions, but if you are still having problems even after incorporating a healthier diet and following your doctor's medical treatment, then you may want to try an elimination diet to determine if you have any food sensitivities or food intolerances.

Among people with food sensitivities, some have always had them, while others have become sensitive to a food by eating one food too often. Sometimes, after you have given your body a break from these food sensitivities, you can add the foods back into your diet as part of a *varied* diet. Variety is key, so we do not overeat those foods again. Others will find that they will have to continue eliminating a food to continue reaping the health benefits and control symptoms.

Gluten is an example of a food Americans could be eating too often, which may be one reason some are becoming sensitive to gluten. In the American diet, we are not getting much variety when it comes to grains. We eat pasta, sandwiches, wraps, pizza, and buns—all of which are made from wheat! So, perhaps we should aim for a variety of whole grains instead of only whole wheat. For one meal, maybe we could eat whole wheat pasta; then we could eat brown rice, quinoa, or oats for the next meal.

Usually, you can eliminate the foods you are sensitive to while simultaneously eating foods that improve your gut health. Once you have healed your gut, many people can add those foods back into their diets. Remember, though, variety is key.

The following are the most common food sensitivities and intolerances:
- Gluten
- Dairy
- Soy
- Yeast
- Corn
- Eggs
- Nuts
- Histamine
- FODMAPs
- Nightshade vegetables
- Cruciferous vegetables

Although science is somewhat conflicting, other possible intolerances that may exasperate ADHD are artificial colors, especially red and yellow, and food additives, such as aspartame and MSG.[130] Fortunately, a whole foods diet will decrease the number of additives and colors consumed.

APPENDIX B
Simple Acts of Kindness Ideas

Going Somewhere and Doing Something
- Before entering any new environment—e.g., work, the grocery store, church, a party, or a park—or even before you get on the internet or social media, pray to God: "God, please help me be loving and kind. Please guide me and help me notice when someone needs help or extra kindness. I know You are here with me right now. Thank you for being with me here in this place and as I am doing this."

Give to Others
- Leave one of your favorite uplifting books at a doctor's office waiting room, in a donation box, or in a local "Little Free Library."
- Put a dollar in a tip jar for no reason.
- Leave a small gift on a neighbor's front door as a happy surprise.
- Make a "Random Acts of Kindness" planner and include local nonprofit agencies and their contacts on your list. Now you have a list on hand whenever you want to help! Call

and email your local agencies and ask them what kinds of donations they need.

- o Examples of local agencies include soup kitchens, nursing homes, hospice, food pantries, homeless shelters, foster care, children's homes, adult daycares, etc.
- Leave some change at a laundry mat.
- Leave a little bag containing some money in an aisle at a store or video drop-off location, so a family can buy snacks to go along with their movie. Add a little note to the bag explaining this Random Act of Kindness.
- Add a note to your kids' or husband's lunches.
- Whenever your school, church, cub scouts, or team holds a service project or donation collection, participate!
- Purchase a gift card at a store, then give it to someone as they walk into the store. We did this for Christmas once. We bought a $50 gift card and then handed it to a mom as she was walking inside the door.
- Have a lemonade stand, cookie stand, or slushy stand and give the money earned to a local charity.
- Call your local school or your child's teacher and ask if they need any school supplies or snacks.
- Say "thank you" to the people who have helped you through life by leaving a gift and a "thank you" note on their front door.
- Leave a quarter on the parking meter. Add a little note to explain this Random Act of Kindness.
- Leave an extra big tip at a restaurant.
- Donate some of your clothes and toys.
- Give water to people on a hot day. Or vice-versa, give them something warm to drink on a cold day.
- Fill a bookbag with school supplies and donate it to "Back the Pack."
- Give away your umbrella to a stranger on a rainy day.

- Leave a little money and a note in random places. Trust God will help the right person find it.
- Donate to a cause or church online.
- Donate to a hospital. Give toys and craft supplies kids can play with while sitting in bed.

Give Your Time

- Volunteer at local nonprofit agencies.
- Make Valentine's, Christmas, or Easter cards and hand-deliver them to the residences at local nursing homes or adult daycares. We did this with Valentine's cards, and the residents loved getting handmade notes hand-delivered from my children.
- Pick up litter in a park. I recommend using gloves or a trash-grabber.
- Buy flowers and hand them out to people on the street or in a park.
- Visit your older or sick family members if you can. They have so much to share!
- Use chalk to write encouraging words on the sidewalk.
- Do chores around the house without having to be asked.
- Send care packages to people you think need one.
- Give blood.
- Draw or color a picture for a friend or family member.
- Volunteer to read to kids at local libraries and bookstores.
- Help someone who is carrying a heavy load of stuff.
- Buy lemonade from a child's lemonade stand.
- Let the kids at a car wash fundraiser wash your vehicle.
- Participate in a local charity walk or run.
- Make a meal for someone. Food is a gift from God. It gives us energy, comforts us, sustains us, and nourishes our bodies. That is why I think giving someone food is the ultimate sign of our love for them.

- Pay for the person behind you in a drive-thru.
- Participate in a local angel tree.
- Participate in your church's donation collection drives. For example, our church has the "Helping Hands" box located in the lobby. This makes donating super simple. We just look in the announcement to see what agency we are helping and what items are being requested, then we add the requested donations to the box! One month, we might be collecting cans; the next month, the church might be asking for winter coats.
- Start your own neighborhood or friends "Helping Hands" box! Leave your box on the porch and get the word out that you are collecting donations. My neighbor's child did this once, and I was amazed by her and the amount of donations she collected. People simply dropped off kids toys at her house, and they took the toys to a children's hospital.
- Babysit for free.
- After eating at a restaurant, stack your plates and wipe the tables. Now the waiter has less to do. This can be super helpful on a busy night!
- If you notice someone with fewer groceries than you in line at the check-out counter, let them go first.
- Give someone you love an unexpected hug.
- Call family members and loved ones just to say "hi."
- Invite friends over for dinner and games.
- Organize a trash pick-up walk in your neighborhood.
- Volunteer at an animal shelter.
- Tutor or read to kids at a local school.
- Volunteer at church.
- Volunteer with Family Promise, or another program to help the homeless. Not all towns have Family Promise, but it is an amazing program! Homeless families stay in local churches while they are working on finding a place to stay. Those local

churches take turns hosting the families. The host church provides dinner for the families, and volunteers spend the night at the church while the families are staying there. Each family has their own room in the church. My family tries to spend the night whenever our church is a host. After we share a meal with these amazing families, my kids love to play with the children in the gym. We usually bring board games and movies to watch right before bed.

Just a Kind Word or Gesture

- Have a Compliments Day: make this a game to see how many compliments you can give out during a day.
- Fill out comment cards or do a quick survey for a restaurant, hotel, or other business. Remember to say something nice even if they didn't have great service. If someone did a good job of helping you, mention them in your comments. I just recently learned what a big deal this is. Not only does doing this brighten the day of the employee who receives the praise, but also it could potentially help someone get a raise or promotion. Management often looks at these comment cards and surveys when making decisions about an employee.
- Send a card to a loved one or friend to let them know you're thinking of them.
- Have an "Ask and Listen" day. Most of us need to listen better, and, sometimes, all someone wants is to be heard. Make an effort to focus on the other person in conversation. Instead of trying to figure out your response to their comment, try to truly listen to what they are saying. Ask questions about them instead of bringing the conversation back to you. Make an effort to talk about the other person's interest.

Social Media

These are so easy and yet so impactful. You don't even have to leave your house to spread love and kindness!

- If a positive thought pops into your head about a post or picture you see as you scroll through your Facebook, Twitter, or Instagram feeds, share it with the person! If we keep the compliment to ourselves, we will miss a chance to lift someone's spirit. Take it a step further and spend some time giving multiple compliments to friends, acquaintances, and strangers.

- Leave a positive and encouraging comment on a blogger or small business's blog post, Facebook page, or Instagram. Even just hitting the "Like" button can help a business. Bloggers and business owners who blog often spend hours perfecting a post. I had never realized how much heart, sweat, and soul a writer puts into a post until I became one. Positively engaging in a post does so much more than lift their spirits. Every like, pin, share, comment, or interaction improves that post's or blog's rankings on their social media accounts. So when you positively engage with someone's post, you are having a huge impact on someone's business without having to purchase a thing!

- Leave a fantastic review! If you love a store, restaurant, business, handmade product, or book, go to one of their social media pages or review page and leave a nice review or comment. Positive reviews can not only make someone's day, but also impact them financially. Think about it. When we buy a product, we love to read the reviews first. The more positive reviews we read, the more likely we will buy that product! If you are reviewing a business, make sure to mention by name any employees who were particularly helpful. This will put a smile on the employees' faces and could also potentially improve their chances of getting a raise or promotion.

Just Plain Fun

- Leave a bag of quarters on an arcade game, a vending machine, or a wishing fountain. Add a little note to the bag explaining this Random Act of Kindness.
- Keep stickers in your pocket or purse. When a child, or mom, looks like they need a little fun distraction, offer a sticker. Be sure to ask the parent for permission before offering the sticker to the child.
- Smile!

APPENDIX C
30-Day Faith-Based Wellness Journal

How to Use This Journal

This thirty-day journal was designed to help you put the practices in this book into action in your daily life. The prompts are the very components I recommend including in your journal as you work to transform your health through faith-based mindfulness and nutrition. The enjoyable, relaxing, and uplifting journal guides your writing, so you are thinking about all the components of this faith-based approach to life.

The following describes each journal prompt:
- Today's Recap
  - Include a short synopsis of your day. Think of all the positive moments of your day. Write about any lessons you learned through your experiences, reading, or Bible studies. Be sure to include any "God moment" stories. You will want to remember those! They're stories about when you notice God working in your life.
- Prayer Moments Today: When Did I Pray Today?
  - In this section, jot down the times you remembered to stop and pray throughout your day.

- My Eating Experience Today: What Foods Did I Eat Today? How Did My Food Nourish Me Today?
  - o Nourishing foods include foods with antioxidants, vitamins, minerals, omega-3s, and other healthy fats. A combination of these nutrient can help promote cognitive function, focus, and alertness; boost moods; reduce anxiety; support the immune system; and reduce the risk of a multitude of chronic diseases. To make sure you are getting these fantastic nutrients in your diet, include foods like vegetables, especially dark leafy greens, fruit, nuts, seeds, whole grains, fish, green tea, and dark chocolate. Limit ultra-processed foods, sweet desserts, packaged pastries, processed meat, fried foods, and refined sugar. For example, when you are writing about your food in your journal, take note of when you have eaten dark leafy greens and be thankful for all the nutrients those greens provide. Keep your journal positive. If you enjoyed a spontaneous family trip to the donut shop, jot down how much you enjoyed your time with your family.
- How Did I Move My Body Today?
  - o Use this section to talk about the ways you exercised your body today. This can be traditional exercise or other physical activity, like gardening or playing outside with your children.
- Thankful Thought for the Day
  - o Being intentional about our thankfulness improves our moods and outlooks on life. So use your journal time to increase your feelings of gratitude.
- How Did I Show Kindness Today?
  - o True health involves the mind, body, and spirit. All are connected. When our spirits are not well, it affects our minds and bodies and vice-versa. Showing kindness

improves the health of our spirits. When you are kind
to others, you will feel better as a whole. So, each day,
take the time to do something kind for someone else
and then record it in your journal.

- My Written Prayer
  - o Take a moment to talk with God in your journal.
    Express your gratitude, tell Him your needs, ask Him
    your questions.

DAY 1

Rejoice always, pray without ceasing, give thanks in all circumstances; for this is the will of God in Christ Jesus for you.
—1 THESSALONIANS 5:16–18 (ESV)

Today's Recap:

Prayer Moments Today: When Did I Pray Today?

My Eating Experience Today: What Foods Did I Eat Today? How Did My Food Nourish Me?

How Did I Move My Body Today?

Thankful Thought for the Day:

How Did I Show Kindness Today?

My Written Prayer

DAY 2

*So whether you eat or drink or whatever you do,
do it all for the glory of God.*
—1 CORINTHIANS 10:31 (NIV)

Today's Recap:

Prayer Moments Today: When Did I Pray Today?

**My Eating Experience Today: What Foods Did I Eat Today?
How Did My Food Nourish Me?**

How Did I Move My Body Today?

Thankful Thought for the Day:

How Did I Show Kindness Today?

My Written Prayer

DAY 3

But the fruit of the Spirit is love, joy, peace, patience,
kindness, goodness, faithfulness, gentleness,
and self-control; against such things is no law.
—GALATIANS 5:22–23 (NIV)

Today's Recap:

Prayer Moments Today: When Did I Pray Today?

My Eating Experience Today: What Foods Did I Eat Today? How Did My Food Nourish Me?

How Did I Move My Body Today?

Thankful Thought for the Day:

How Did I Show Kindness Today?

My Written Prayer

DAY 4

Then God said, "I give you every seed-bearing plant
on the face of the whole earth and every tree that has
fruit with seed in it. They will be yours for food."
—GENESIS 1:29 (NIV)

Today's Recap:

Prayer Moments Today: When Did I Pray Today?

My Eating Experience Today: What Foods Did I Eat Today?
How Did My Food Nourish Me?

How Did I Move My Body Today?

Thankful Thought for the Day:

How Did I Show Kindness Today?

My Written Prayer

DAY 5

He gives food to every creature. His love endures forever.
—PSALM 136:25 (NIV)

Today's Recap:

Prayer Moments Today: When Did I Pray Today?

**My Eating Experience Today: What Foods Did I Eat Today?
How Did My Food Nourish Me?**

How Did I Move My Body Today?

Thankful Thought for the Day:

How Did I Show Kindness Today?

My Written Prayer

DAY 6

Be still and know that I am God.
—PSALM 46:10 (NIV)

Today's Recap:

Prayer Moments Today: When Did I Pray Today?

My Eating Experience Today: What Foods Did I Eat Today? How Did My Food Nourish Me?

How Did I Move My Body Today?

Thankful Thought for the Day:

How Did I Show Kindness Today?

My Written Prayer

DAY 7

Do not be anxious about anything,
but in every situation, by prayer and petition,
with thanksgiving, present your requests to God.
—PHILIPPIANS 4:6 (NIV)

Today's Recap:

Prayer Moments Today: When Did I Pray Today?

My Eating Experience Today: What Foods Did I Eat Today? How Did My Food Nourish Me?

How Did I Move My Body Today?

Thankful Thought for the Day:

How Did I Show Kindness Today?

My Written Prayer

DAY 8

Devote yourselves to prayer, being watchful and thankful.
—COLOSSIANS 4:2 (NIV)

Today's Recap:

Prayer Moments Today: When Did I Pray Today?

**My Eating Experience Today: What Foods Did I Eat Today?
How Did My Food Nourish Me?**

How Did I Move My Body Today?

Thankful Thought for the Day:

How Did I Show Kindness Today?

My Written Prayer

DAY 9

So whatever you wish that others would do to you, do also to them, for this is the Law and the Prophets.
—MATTHEW 7:12 (ESV)

Today's Recap:

Prayer Moments Today: When Did I Pray Today?

My Eating Experience Today: What Foods Did I Eat Today? How Did My Food Nourish Me?

How Did I Move My Body Today?

Thankful Thought for the Day:

How Did I Show Kindness Today?

My Written Prayer

DAY 10

He said to his disciples, "Why are you so afraid?
Do you still have no faith?"
—MARK 4:40 (NIV)

Today's Recap:

Prayer Moments Today: When Did I Pray Today?

My Eating Experience Today: What Foods Did I Eat Today?
How Did My Food Nourish Me?

How Did I Move My Body Today?

Thankful Thought for the Day:

How Did I Show Kindness Today?

My Written Prayer

DAY 11

After the earthquake came a fire, but the Lord was not in the fire.
And after the fire came a gentle whisper.
—1 KINGS 19:12 (NIV)

Today's Recap:

Prayer Moments Today: When Did I Pray Today?

My Eating Experience Today: What Foods Did I Eat Today?
How Did My Food Nourish Me?

How Did I Move My Body Today?

Thankful Thought for the Day:

How Did I Show Kindness Today?

My Written Prayer

DAY 12

For God so loved the world that he gave his one and only Son,
that whoever believes in him shall not perish but have eternal life.
—JOHN 3:16 (NIV)

Today's Recap:

Prayer Moments Today: When Did I Pray Today?

My Eating Experience Today: What Foods Did I Eat Today?
How Did My Food Nourish Me?

How Did I Move My Body Today?

Thankful Thought for the Day:

How Did I Show Kindness Today?

My Written Prayer

DAY 13

Since we are living by the Spirit, let us follow the
Spirit's leading in every part of our lives.
—GALATIANS 5:25 (NLT)

Today's Recap:

Prayer Moments Today: When Did I Pray Today?

My Eating Experience Today: What Foods Did I Eat Today?
How Did My Food Nourish Me?

How Did I Move My Body Today?

Thankful Thought for the Day:

How Did I Show Kindness Today?

My Written Prayer

DAY 14

*And we know that for those who love God all
things work together for good, for those who are
called according to his purpose.*
—ROMANS 8:28 (ESV)

Today's Recap:

Prayer Moments Today: When Did I Pray Today?

**My Eating Experience Today: What Foods Did I Eat Today?
How Did My Food Nourish Me?**

How Did I Move My Body Today?

Thankful Thought for the Day:

How Did I Show Kindness Today?

My Written Prayer

DAY 15

"Have I not commanded you? Be strong and courageous.
Do not be frightened, and do not be dismayed,
for the Lord your God is with you wherever you go."
—Joshua 1:9 (ESV)

Today's Recap:

Prayer Moments Today: When Did I Pray Today?

My Eating Experience Today: What Foods Did I Eat Today?
How Did My Food Nourish Me?

How Did I Move My Body Today?

Thankful Thought for the Day:

How Did I Show Kindness Today?

My Written Prayer

DAY 16

With God all things are possible.
—MATTHEW 19:26 (NIV)

Today's Recap:

Prayer Moments Today: When Did I Pray Today?

**My Eating Experience Today: What Foods Did I Eat Today?
How Did My Food Nourish Me?**

How Did I Move My Body Today?

Thankful Thought for the Day:

How Did I Show Kindness Today?

My Written Prayer

DAY 17

Great is our Lord, and abundant in power;
his understanding is beyond measure.
—PSALM 147:5 (ESV)

Today's Recap:

Prayer Moments Today: When Did I Pray Today?

My Eating Experience Today: What Foods Did I Eat Today?
How Did My Food Nourish Me?

How Did I Move My Body Today?

Thankful Thought for the Day:

How Did I Show Kindness Today?

My Written Prayer

DAY 18

But God demonstrates his own love for us in this:
While we were still sinners, Christ died for us.
—ROMANS 5:8 (NIV)

Today's Recap:

Prayer Moments Today: When Did I Pray Today?

My Eating Experience Today: What Foods Did I Eat Today?
How Did My Food Nourish Me?

How Did I Move My Body Today?

Thankful Thought for the Day:

How Did I Show Kindness Today?

My Written Prayer

DAY 19

And the peace of God, which surpasses all comprehension, will guard your hearts and minds in Christ Jesus.
—Philippians 4:7 (New American Standard Bible)

Today's Recap:

Prayer Moments Today: When Did I Pray Today?

My Eating Experience Today: What Foods Did I Eat Today? How Did My Food Nourish Me?

How Did I Move My Body Today?

Thankful Thought for the Day:

How Did I Show Kindness Today?

My Written Prayer

DAY 20

And he said to them, "Come away by yourselves to a secluded place and rest a little while." For there were many people coming and going, and they did not even have time to eat.
—MARK 6:31 (NASB)

Today's Recap:

Prayer Moments Today: When Did I Pray Today?

My Eating Experience Today: What Foods Did I Eat Today? How Did My Food Nourish Me?

How Did I Move My Body Today?

Thankful Thought for the Day:

How Did I Show Kindness Today?

My Written Prayer

DAY 21

So do not worry about tomorrow; for tomorrow will worry about itself. Each day has enough trouble of its own.
—MATTHEW 6:34 (NASB)

Today's Recap:

Prayer Moments Today: When Did I Pray Today?

My Eating Experience Today: What Foods Did I Eat Today? How Did My Food Nourish Me?

How Did I Move My Body Today?

Thankful Thought for the Day:

How Did I Show Kindness Today?

My Written Prayer

DAY 22

Come to me, all who are weary and burdened,
and I will give you rest.
—MATTHEW 11:28 (NASB)

Today's Recap:

Prayer Moments Today: When Did I Pray Today?

My Eating Experience Today: What Foods Did I Eat Today?
How Did My Food Nourish Me?

How Did I Move My Body Today?

Thankful Thought for the Day:

How Did I Show Kindness Today?

My Written Prayer

DAY 23

*And he answered, "You shall love the Lord your God with all
your heart, and with all your soul, and with all your strength,
and with all your mind; and your neighbor as yourself."*
—LUKE 10:27 (NIV)

Today's Recap:

Prayer Moments Today: When Did I Pray Today?

**My Eating Experience Today: What Foods Did I Eat Today?
How Did My Food Nourish Me?**

How Did I Move My Body Today?

Thankful Thought for the Day:

How Did I Show Kindness Today?

My Written Prayer

DAY 24

But I say to you who hear, love your enemies,
do good to those who hate you.
—LUKE 6:27 (NASB)

Today's Recap:

Prayer Moments Today: When Did I Pray Today?

My Eating Experience Today: What Foods Did I Eat Today?
How Did My Food Nourish Me?

How Did I Move My Body Today?

Thankful Thought for the Day:

How Did I Show Kindness Today?

My Written Prayer

DAY 25

Treat people the same way you want them to treat you.
—LUKE 6:31 (NASB)

Today's Recap:

Prayer Moments Today: When Did I Pray Today?

My Eating Experience Today: What Foods Did I Eat Today? How Did My Food Nourish Me?

How Did I Move My Body Today?

Thankful Thought for the Day:

How Did I Show Kindness Today?

My Written Prayer

DAY 26

Go, eat your food with gladness, and drink your wine with a joyful heart, for God has already approved what you do.
—ECCLESIASTES 9:7 (NIV)

Today's Recap:

Prayer Moments Today: When Did I Pray Today?

My Eating Experience Today: What Foods Did I Eat Today? How Did My Food Nourish Me?

How Did I Move My Body Today?

Thankful Thought for the Day:

How Did I Show Kindness Today?

My Written Prayer

DAY 27

How precious is your loving kindness, O God! And the
children of men take refuge in the shadow of your wings.
—PSALM 36:7 (AMPLIFIED BIBLE)

Today's Recap:

Prayer Moments Today: When Did I Pray Today?

My Eating Experience Today: What Foods Did I Eat Today?
How Did My Food Nourish Me?

How Did I Move My Body Today?

Thankful Thought for the Day:

How Did I Show Kindness Today?

My Written Prayer

DAY 28

Gracious words are a honeycomb,
sweet to the soul and healing to the bones.
—Proverbs 16:24 (NASB)

Today's Recap:

Prayer Moments Today: When Did I Pray Today?

My Eating Experience Today: What Foods Did I Eat Today?
How Did My Food Nourish Me?

How Did I Move My Body Today?

Thankful Thought for the Day:

How Did I Show Kindness Today?

My Written Prayer

DAY 29

But now faith, hope, and love remain, these three;
but the greatest of these is love.
—1 Corinthians 13:13 (NASB)

Today's Recap:

Prayer Moments Today: When Did I Pray Today?

My Eating Experience Today: What Foods Did I Eat Today?
How Did My Food Nourish Me?

How Did I Move My Body Today?

Thankful Thought for the Day:

How Did I Show Kindness Today?

My Written Prayer

DAY 30

We love, because he first loved us.
—1 JOHN 4:19 (NASB)

Today's Recap:

Prayer Moments Today: When Did I Pray Today?

My Eating Experience Today: What Foods Did I Eat Today? How Did My Food Nourish Me?

How Did I Move My Body Today?

Thankful Thought for the Day:

How Did I Show Kindness Today?

My Written Prayer

ENDNOTES

1 Thida Tabucanon, Jennifer Wilcox, and W. H. Wilson Tang, "Does Weight Loss Improve Clinical Outcomes in Overweight and Obese Patients with Heart Failure?" *Current Diabetes Reports* 20, no. 75 (2020), https://doi.org/10.1007/s11892-020-01367-z; Sankar D. Navaneenthan et al., "Weight Loss Interventions in Chronic Kidney Disease: A Systematic Review and Meta-analysis," *Clinical Journal of the American Society of Nephrology* 4, no. 10 (2009): 1565–1574, https://doi.org/10.2215/cjn.02250409; William T. Cefalu, "Achieving Type 2 Diabetes Remission Through Weight Loss," *Diabetes Discoveries & Practice Blog*, National Institute of Diabetes and Digestive and Kidney Diseases, September 30, 2020, https://www.niddk.nih.gov/health-information/professionals/diabetes-discoveries-practice/achieving-type-2-diabetes-remission-through-weight-loss; Pascal Richette et al., "Benefits of Massive Weight Loss on Symptoms, Systemic Inflammation and Cartilage Turnover in Obese Patients With Knee Osteoarthritis," *BMJ Journals* 70, no. 1 (2011): 139–144, https://doi.org/10.1136/ard.2010.134015; Daniel P. Schauer et al., "Association Between Weight Loss and the Risk of Cancer After Bariatric Surgery," *The Obesity Society* 25, no. S2 (2017): S52–7, https://doi.org/10.1002/oby.22002; and Jody A. Vogel et al., "Reduction in Predicted Coronary Heart Disease Risk After Substantial Weight Reduction After Bariatric Surgery," *The American Journal of Cardiology* 99, no. 2 (2007): 222–6, https://doi.org/10.1016/j.amjcard.2006.08.017.

2 J. Aust and T. Bradshaw, "Mindfulness Interventions for Psychosis: A Systematic Review of the Literature," *Journal of Psychiatric and Mental Health Nursing* 24, no. 1 (2016): 69–83, https://doi.org/10.1111/jpm.12357; Christine E. Cherpak, "Mindful Eating: A Review of How the Stress-digestion Mindfulness Triad May Modulate and Improve Gastrointestinal and Digestive Function," *Integrative Medicine* 18, no. 4 (2019): 48–53, https://pubmed.ncbi.nlm.nih.gov/32549835/; "Mindful Eating," The Nutrition Source, Harvard School of Public Health, posted September 18, 2020, https://www.hsph.harvard.edu/nutritionsource/mindful-eating/; Joseph B. Nelson, "Mindful Eating: The Art of Presence While You Eat," *Diabetes Spectrum* 30, no. 3 (2017): 171–4, https://doi.org/10.2337/ds17-0015; and Clara Strauss et al., "Mindfulness-Based Interventions for People Diagnosed with a Current Episode of an Anxiety or Depressive Disorder: A Meta-Analysis of Randomised Controlled Trials," *PLoS ONE* 9, no. 4 (2014): e96110, https://doi.org/10.1371/journal.pone.0096110.

3   Moisés E. Bauer and Antonio L. Teixeira, "Inflammation in Psychiatric Disorders: What Comes First?" *Annals of the New York Academy of Sciences* 1437, no. 1 (2018): 57–67, https://doi.org/10.1111/nyas.13712; Alison C. Bested, Alan C. Logan, and Eva M. Selhub, "Intestinal Microbiota, Probiotics and Mental Health: From Metchnikoff to Modern Advances: Part II – Contemporary Contextual Research," *Gut Pathogens* 5, no. 1 (2013): 3, https://doi.org/10.1186/1757-4749-5-3; Cherpak, "Mindful Eating"; Dianne Rishikof, *Health Takes Guts,* (self-published, 2018), Kindle; and Neil Schneiderman, Gail Ironson, and Scott D. Siegel, "Stress and Health: Psychological, Behavioral, and Biological Determinants," *Annual Review of Clinical Psychology* 1, no. 1 (2005): 607–28, https://doi.org/10.1146/annurev.clinpsy.1.102803.144141.

4   Cherpak, "Mindful Eating"; and Clara Strauss et al., "Mindfulness-Based Interventions."

5   Cherpak, "Mindful Eating"; and Rishikof, *Health Takes Guts.*

6   Michael C. Abt et al., "Commensal Bacteria Calibrate the Activation Threshold of Innate Antiviral Immunity," *Immunity* 37, no. 1 (2012): 158–70, https://doi.org/10.1016/j.immuni.2012.04.011; Ghodarz Akkasheh et al., "Clinical and Metabolic Response to Probiotic Administration in Patients with Major Depressive Disorder: A Randomized, Double-blind, Placebo-controlled Trial," *Nutrition* 32, no. 3 (2016): 315–20, https://doi.org/10.1016/j.nut.2015.09.003; Bested, Logan, and Selhub, "Intestinal Microbiota"; Stephanie Bull-Larsen and M. Hasan Mohajeri, "The Potential Influence of the Bacterial Microbiome on the Development and Progression of ADHD," *Nutrients* 11, no. 11 (2019): 2805, https://doi.org/10.3390/nu11112805; Cherpak, "Mindful Eating"; Rashmi R. Das, Meenu Singh, and Shafiq Nusrat, "Probiotics for Prevention or Treatment of Asthma," *Chest* 138, no. 4 (2010): 307A, https://doi.org/10.1378/chest.9485; C. Bernard Gesch et al., "Influence of Supplementary Vitamins, Minerals and Essential Fatty Acids on the Antisocial Behaviour of Young Adult Prisoners," *British Journal of Psychiatry* 181, no. 1 (2002): 22–8, https://doi.org/10.1192/bjp.181.1.22; Ruixue Huang, Ke Wang, and Jianan Hu, "Effect of Probiotics on Depression: A Systematic Review and Meta-Analysis of Randomized Controlled Trials," *Nutrients* 8, no. 8 (2016): 483, https://doi.org/10.3390/nu8080483; Osamu Kanauchi et al., "Probiotics and Paraprobiotics in Viral Infection: Clinical Application and Effects on the Innate and Acquired Immune Systems," *Current Pharmaceutical Design* 24, no. 6 (2018): 710–7, https://doi.org/10.2174/1381612824666180116163411; En-Jin Kang et al., "The Effect of Probiotics on Prevention of Common Cold: A Meta-Analysis of Randomized Controlled Trial Studies," *Korean Journal of Family Medicine* 34, no. 1 (2013): 2, https://doi.org/10.4082/kjfm.2013.34.1.2; Hojka Gregoric Kumperscak et al., "A Pilot Randomized Control Trial with the Probiotic Strain *Lactobacillus Rhamnosus* GG (LGG) in ADHD: Children and Adolescents Report Better Health-related Quality of Life," *Frontiers in Psychiatry* 11, (2020): 181, https://doi.org/10.3389/fpsyt.2020.00181; Rikke Pilmann Laursen and Iva Hojsak, "Probiotics for Respiratory Tract Infections in Children Attending Day Care Centers-A Systematic Review," *European Journal of Pediatrics* 177, no. 7 (2018): 979–94, https://doi.org/10.1007/s00431-018-3167-1; Clara S. C. Lee et al., "The Effectiveness of Mindfulness-based Intervention in Attention on Individuals with ADHD: A Systematic Review," *Hong Kong Journal of Occupational Therapy* 30, no. 1 (2017): 33–41, https://doi.org/10.1016/j.hkjot.2017.05.001; L. Lehtoranta, A. Pitkäranta, and R. Korpela, "Probiotics in Respiratory Virus Infections," *European Journal of Clinical Microbiology & Infectious Diseases* 33, no. 8 (2014): 1289–302, https://doi.org/10.1007/s10096-014-2086-y; Stephanie Louise et al., "Mindfulness- and Acceptance-based Interventions for Psychosis: Our Current Understanding and a

Meta-Analysis," *Schizophrenia Research* 192, (2018): 57–63, https://doi.org/10.1016/j.schres.2017.05.023; Kassem Makki et al., "The Impact of Dietary Fiber on Gut Microbiota in Host Health and Disease," *Cell Host & Microbe* 23, no. 6 (2018): 705–15, https://doi.org/10.1016/j.chom.2018.05.012; Kalai Mathee et al., "The Gut Microbiome and Neuropsychiatric Disorders: Implications for Attention Deficit Hyperactivity Disorder (ADHD)," *Journal of Medical Microbiology* 69, no. 1 (2020): 14–24, https://doi.org/10.1099/jmm.0.001112; Michaël Messaoudi et al., "Beneficial Psychological Effects of a Probiotic Formulation (Lactobacillus Helveticusr0052 Andbifidobacterium Longumr0175) in Healthy Human Volunteers," *Gut Microbes* 2, no. 4 (2011): 256–61, https://doi.org/10.4161/gmic.2.4.16108; Ali Akbar Mohammadi et al., "The Effects of Probiotics on Mental Health and Hypothalamic–Pituitary–Adrenal Axis: A Randomized, Double-blind, Placebo-controlled Trial in Petrochemical Workers," *Nutritional Neuroscience* 19, no. 9 (2015): 387–95, https://doi.org/10.1179/1476830515y.0000000023; Joseph B. Nelson, "Mindful Eating: The Art of Presence While You Eat," *Diabetes Spectrum* 30, no. 3 (2017): 171–4, https://doi.org/10.2337/ds17-0015; Qin Xiang Ng et al., "A Systematic Review of the Role of Prebiotics and Probiotics in Autism Spectrum Disorders," *Medicina* 55, no. 5 (2019): 129, https://doi.org/10.3390/medicina55050129; Anna Pärtty et al., "A Possible Link Between Early Probiotic Intervention and the Risk of Neuropsychiatric Disorders Later in Childhood: A Randomized Trial," *Pediatric Research* 77, no. 6 (2015): 823–8, https://doi.org/10.1038/pr.2015.51; Rishikof, *Health Takes Guts*; Neil Schneiderman, Gail Ironson, and Scott D. Siegel, "Stress and Health: Psychological, Behavioral, and Biological Determinants," *Annual Review of Clinical Psychology* 1, no. 1 (2005): 607–28, https://doi.org/10.1146/annurev.clinpsy.1.102803.144141; Sanaa Y. Shaaban et al., "The Role of Probiotics in Children with Autism Spectrum Disorder: A Prospective, Open-Label Study," *Nutritional Neuroscience* 21, no. 9 (2017): 676–81, https://doi.org/10.1080/1028415x.2017.1347746; Jia-Ling Sheng et al., "The Effects of Mindfulness Meditation on Hallucination and Delusion in Severe Schizophrenia Patients with More Than 20 Years' Medical History," *CNS Neuroscience & Therapeutics* 25, no. 1 (2018): 147–50, https://doi.org/10.1111/cns.13067; Clara Strauss et al., "Mindfulness-Based Interventions"; M. Takada et al., "Probiotic Lactobacillus Casei Strain Shirota Relieves Stress-associated Symptoms by Modulating the Gut-Brain Interaction in Human and Animal Models," *Neurogastroenterology & Motility* 28, no. 7 (2016): 1027–36, https://doi.org/10.1111/nmo.12804; Yizhong Wang et al., "Probiotics for Prevention and Treatment of Respiratory Tract Infections in Children," *Medicine* 95, no. 31 (2016): e4509, https://doi.org/10.1097/md.0000000000004509; Jiaming Xue, Yun Zhang, and Ying Huang, "A Meta-Analytic Investigation of the Impact of Mindfulness-based Interventions on ADHD Symptoms," *Medicine* 98, no. 23 (2019): e15957, https://doi.org/10.1097/md.0000000000015957; and Marilyn Haugen and Doug Cook, 175 *Superfood Blender Recipes: Using Your NutriBullet* (Ontario: Robert Rose, 2016).

7 Maggie Moon, *The MIND Diet: A Scientific Approach to Enhancing Brain Function and Helping Prevent Alzheimer's and Dementia*, 1st ed. (California: Ulysses Press, 2016).

8 ——, *The MIND Diet*.

9 María A. Puertollano et al., "Dietary Antioxidants: Immunity and Host Defense," *Current Topics in Medicinal Chemistry* 11, no. 14 (2011): 1752–66, https://doi.org/10.2174/156802611796235107; Muhammad Abdullah et al., "The Effectiveness of Omega-3 Supplementation in Reducing ADHD Associated Symptoms in Children as Measured by the Conners' Rating Scales: A Systematic Review of Randomized

Controlled Trials," *Journal of Psychiatric Research* 110 (2019): 64–73, https://doi. org/10.1016/j.jpsychires.2018.12.002; Shahieda Adams et al., "Relationship Between Serum Omega-3 Fatty Acid and Asthma Endpoints," *International Journal of Environmental Research and Public Health* 16, no. 1 (2018) 43, https://doi.org/10.3390/ ijerph16010043; Lourdes Alvarez-Arellano et al., "Antioxidants as a Potential Target Against Inflammation and Oxidative Stress in Attention-deficit/Hyperactivity Disorder," *Antioxidants* 9, no. 2 (2020): 176, https://doi.org/10.3390/antiox9020176; Bradley M. Appelhans et al., "Depression Severity, Diet Quality, and Physical Activity in Women with Obesity and Depression," *Journal of the Academy of Nutrition and Dietetics* 112, no. 5 (2012): 693–8, https://doi.org/10.1016/j.jand.2012.02.006; A. Bendich, "Physiological Role of Antioxidants in the Immune System," *Journal of Dairy Science* 76, no. 9 (1993): 2789–94, https://doi.org/10.3168/jds.s0022-0302(93)77617-1; Jose A. Castro-Rodriguez and Luis Garcia-Marcos, "What Are the Effects of a Mediterranean Diet on Allergies and Asthma in Children?" *Frontiers in Pediatrics* 5, (2017a): 72, https://doi.org/10.3389/fped.2017.00072; Ruth E. Cooper et al., "The Effect of Omega-3 Polyunsaturated Fatty Acid Supplementation on Emotional Dysregulation, Oppositional Behaviour and Conduct Problems in ADHD: A Systematic Review and Meta-Analysis," *Journal of Affective Disorders* 190, (2016): 474–82, https://doi. org/10.1016/j.jad.2015.09.053; Maria Fernandes, David M. Mutch, and Francesco Leri, "The Relationship Between Fatty Acids and Different Depression-related Brain Regions, and Their Potential Role as Biomarkers of Response to Antidepressants," *Nutrients* 9, no. 3 (2017): 298, https://doi.org/10.3390/nu9030298; Mary A. Fristad et al., "Pilot Randomized Controlled Trial of Omega-3 and Individual Family Psychoeducational Psychotherapy for Children and Adolescents with Depression," *Journal of Clinical Child & Adolescent Psychology* 48, sup. 1 (2016): S105–18, https://doi.org/10.1080/1537441 6.2016.1233500; Medhavi Gautam et al., "Role of Antioxidants in Generalized Anxiety Disorder and Depression," *Indian Journal of Psychiatry* 54, no. 3 (2012): 244, https:// doi.org/10.4103/0019-5545.102424; Fernando Gómez-Pinilla, "Brain Foods: The Effects of Nutrients on Brain Function," *Nature Reviews Neuroscience* 9, no. 7 (2008): 568–78, https://doi.org/10.1038/nrn2421; Olivia M. Guillin et al., "Selenium, Selenoproteins and Viral Infection," *Nutrients* 11, no. 9 (2019): 2101, https://doi.org/10.3390/ nu11092101; Anita L. Hansen et al., "Reduced Anxiety in Forensic Inpatients After a Long-term Intervention with Atlantic Salmon," *Nutrients* 6, no. 12 (2014): 5405–18, https://doi.org/10.3390/nu6125405; D. Hewedi, G. Mostafa, and E. M. A. N. El Hadidi, "Oxidative Stress in Egyptian Children with Autism: Relation to Autoimmunity," *European Psychiatry* 30, (2015): 807, https://doi.org/10.1016/s0924- 9338(15)30628-3; Qingyi Huang et al., "Linking What We Eat to Our Mood: A Review of Diet, Dietary Antioxidants, and Depression," *Antioxidants* 8, no. 9 (2019): 376, https://doi.org/10.3390/antiox8090376; Felice N. Jacka et al., "A Randomised Controlled Trial of Dietary Improvement for Adults with Major Depression (The 'SMILES' Trial)," *BMC Medicine* 15, no. 1 (2017): 23, https://doi.org/10.1186/ s12916-017-0791-y; Wilhelmina Kalt et al., "Recent Research on the Health Benefits of Blueberries and Their Anthocyanins," *Advances in Nutrition* 11, no. 2 (2020): 224–36, https://doi.org/10.1093/advances/nmz065; Sundus Khalid et al., "Effects of Acute Blueberry Flavonoids on Mood in Children and Young Adults," *Nutrients* 9, no. 2 (2017): 158, https://doi.org/10.3390/nu9020158; Sarah Klemm, "Support Your Health with Nutrition," EatRight.Org, Academy of Nutrition and Dietetics, published December 9, 2019, reviewed April 2020, https://www.eatright.org/health/wellness/ preventing-illness/support-your-health-with-nutrition; Yuzo Kodama et al., "Antioxidant

Nutrients in Plasma of Japanese Patients with Chronic Obstructive Pulmonary Disease, Asthma-COPD Overlap Syndrome and Bronchial Asthma," *The Clinical Respiratory Journal* 11, no. 6 (2016): 915–24, https://doi.org/10.1111/crj.12436; Undine E. Lang et al., "Nutritional Aspects of Depression," *Cellular Physiology and Biochemistry* 37, no. 3 (2015): 1029–43, https://doi.org/10.1159/000430229; Emma K. Larkin et al., "New Risk Factors for Adult-Onset Incident Asthma. A Nested Case-Control Study of Host Antioxidant Defense," *American Journal of Respiratory and Critical Care Medicine* 191, no. 1 (2015): 45–53, https://doi.org/10.1164/rccm.201405-0948oc; Ye Li et al., "Dietary Patterns and Depression Risk: A Meta-Analysis," *Psychiatry Research* 253, (2017): 373–82, https://doi.org/10.1016/j.psychres.2017.04.020; Lars Lien et al., "Consumption of Soft Drinks and Hyperactivity, Mental Distress, and Conduct Problems Among Adolescents in Oslo, Norway," *American Journal of Public Health* 96, no. 10 (2006): 1815–20, https://doi.org/10.2105/ajph.2004.059477; Pedro V. S. Magalhães et al., "Antioxidant Treatments for Schizophrenia," *Cochrane Database of Systematic Reviews* 2, (2016): CD008919, https://doi.org/10.1002/14651858.cd008919.pub2; Makki et al., "Dietary Fiber"; Thamilarasan Manivasagam et al., "Role of Oxidative Stress and Antioxidants in Autism," *Advances in Neurobiology* 24, (2020): 193–206, https://doi.org/10.1007/978-3-030-30402-7_7; Takako Miki et al., "Dietary Fiber Intake and Depressive Symptoms in Japanese Employees: The Furukawa Nutrition and Health Study," *Nutrition* 32, no. 5 (2016): 584–9, https://doi.org/10.1016/j.nut.2015.11.014; Catherine M. Milte et al., "Eicosapentaenoic and Docosahexaenoic Acids, Cognition, and Behavior in Children with Attention-Deficit/Hyperactivity Disorder: A Randomized Controlled Trial," *Nutrition* 28, no. 6 (2012): 670–7, https://doi.org/10.1016/j.nut.2011.12.009; Moon, *The MIND Diet*; Kristen Chang, "Nutrition & Immune Health," Virginia Academy of Nutrition and Dietetics, published January 14, 2016, https://eatrightvirginia.org/nutrition-immune-health/; Joel T. Nigg and Kathleen Holton, "Restriction and Elimination Diets in ADHD Treatment," *Child and Adolescent Psychiatric Clinics of North America* 23, no. 4 (2014): 937–53, https://doi.org/10.1016/j.chc.2014.05.010; Adrienne O'Neil et al., "Relationship Between Diet and Mental Health in Children and Adolescents: A Systematic Review," *American Journal of Public Health* 104, no. 10 (2014): e31–42, https://doi.org/10.2105/ajph.2014.302110; Rachelle S. Opie et al., "A Modified Mediterranean Dietary Intervention for Adults with Major Depression: Dietary Protocol and Feasibility Data from the SMILES Trial," *Nutritional Neuroscience* 21, no. 7 (2017): 487–501, https://doi.org/10.1080/1028415x.2017.1312841; Shae E. Quirk et al., "The Association Between Diet Quality, Dietary Patterns and Depression in Adults: A Systematic Review," *BMC Psychiatry* 13, no. 1 (2013): 175, https://doi.org/10.1186/1471-244x-13-175; Alejandra Ríos-Hernández et al., "The Mediterranean Diet and ADHD in Children and Adolescents," *Pediatrics* 139, no. 2 (2017): e20162027, https://doi.org/10.1542/peds.2016-2027; Rishikof, *Health Takes Guts*; Faezeh Saghafian et al., "Fruit and Vegetable Consumption and Risk of Depression: Accumulative Evidence from an Updated Systematic Review and Meta-Analysis of Epidemiological Studies," *British Journal of Nutrition* 119, no. 10 (2018): 1087–101, https://doi.org/10.1017/s0007114518000697; Samina Salim, Gaurav Chugh, and Mohammad Asghar, "Inflammation in Anxiety," *Advances in Protein Chemistry and Structural Biology* 88, (2012): 1–25, https://doi.org/10.1016/b978-0-12-398314-5.00001-5; Jerome Sarris et al., "Nutritional Medicine as Mainstream in Psychiatry," *The Lancet Psychiatry* 2, no. 3 (2015): 271–4, https://doi.org/10.1016/s2215-0366(14)00051-0; Vaughan S. Somerville, Andrea J. Braakhuis, and Will G. Hopkins, "Effect of Flavonoids on Upper Respiratory Tract Infections and Immune Function: A Systematic Review and

Meta-Analysis," *Advances in Nutrition* 7, no. 3 (2016): 488–97, https://doi.org/10.3945/an.115.010538; Isobel Stoodley et al., "Higher Omega-3 Index Is Associated with Better Asthma Control and Lower Medication Dose: A Cross-sectional Study," *Nutrients* 12, no. 1 (2019): 74, https://doi.org/10.3390/nu12010074; Kuan-Pin Su, Yutaka Matsuoka, and Chi-Un Pae, "Omega-3 Polyunsaturated Fatty Acids in Prevention of Mood and Anxiety Disorders," *Clinical Psychopharmacology and Neuroscience* 13, no. 2 (2015): 129–37, https://doi.org/10.9758/cpn.2015.13.2.129; Annelies A. Verlaet et al., "Rationale for Dietary Antioxidant Treatment of ADHD," *Nutrients* 10, no. 4 (2018): 405, https://doi.org/10.3390/nu10040405; K. C. Wright, "Clinical Nutrition: Beyond Food and Mood," *Today's Dietitian* 21, no. 7 (2019): 10, https://www.todaysdietitian.com/newarchives/0719p10.shtml; Yang Yang et al., "Association Between Dietary Fiber and Lower Risk of All-Cause Mortality: A Meta-Analysis of Cohort Studies," *American Journal of Epidemiology* 181, no. 2 (2015): 83–91, https://doi.org/10.1093/aje/kwu257; and Andrea S. Young et al., "Psychoeducational Psychotherapy and Omega-3 Supplementation Improve Co-Occurring Behavioral Problems in Youth with Depression: Results from a Pilot RCT," *Journal of Abnormal Child Psychology* 45, no. 5 (2016): 1025–37, https://doi.org/10.1007/s10802-016-0203-3.
10 Ríos-Hernández et al., "The Mediterranean Diet."
11 N. A. Mikirova et al., "Metabolic Correction for Attention Deficit/Hyperactivity Disorder: A Biochemical-physiological Therapeutic Approach," *Functional Foods in Health and Disease* 3, no. 1 (2013): 1, https://doi.org/10.31989/ffhd.v3i1.67.
12 ——, "Metabolic Correction"; and Pablo Roman et al., "A Pilot Randomized Controlled Trial to Explore Cognitive and Emotional Effects of Probiotics in Fibromyalgia," *Scientific Reports* 8, no. 1 (2018): 10965, https://doi.org/10.1038/s41598-018-29388-5.
13 Castro-Rodriguez and Garcia-Marcos, "Effects of a Mediterranean Diet."
14 Laurent Guilleminault et al., "Diet and Asthma: Is It Time to Adapt Our Message?" *Nutrients* 9, no. 11 (2017): 1227, https://doi.org/10.3390/nu9111227.
15 Kodama et al., "Antioxidant Nutrients"; and Larkin et al., "New Risk Factors."
16 Maria Chiara Mentella et al., "Cancer and Mediterranean Diet: A Review," *Nutrients* 11, no. 9 (2019): 2059, https://doi.org/10.3390/nu11092059.
17 Jacka et al., "Controlled Trial."
18 "Food Guidelines," Blue Zones, September 7, 2020, https://www.bluezones.com/recipes/food-guidelines/.
19 Puertollano et al., "Dietary Antioxidants"; Alvarez-Arellano et al., "Potential Target"; Bauer and Teixeira, "Inflammation in Psychiatric Disorders"; Bendich, "Physiological Role"; Daria Brambilla et al., "The Role of Antioxidant Supplement in Immune System, Neoplastic, and Neurodegenerative Disorders: A Point of View for an Assessment of the Risk/Benefit Profile," *Nutrition Journal* 7, no. 1 (2008): 29, https://doi.org/10.1186/1475-2891-7-29; James R. Cerhan et al., "Antioxidant Micronutrients and Risk of Rheumatoid Arthritis in a Cohort of Older Women," *American Journal of Epidemiology* 157, no. 4 (2003): 345–54, https://doi.org/10.1093/aje/kwf205; Wright, "Beyond Food and Mood"; Andrea Deledda et al., "Diet-derived Antioxidants and Their Role in Inflammation, Obesity and Gut Microbiota Modulation," *Antioxidants* 10, no. 5 (2021): 708, https://doi.org/10.3390/antiox10050708; Melissa Eaton, Joseph Firth, and Jerome Sarris, "Nutrition and Mental Health—How the Food We Eat Can Affect Our Mood," *Frontiers for Young Minds* 8, (2020): 115, https://doi.org/10.3389/frym.2020.00115; Daisuke Furushima, Kazuki Ide, and Hiroshi Yamada, "Effect of Tea Catechins on Influenza Infection and the Common Cold with a Focus

on Epidemiological/Clinical Studies," *Molecules* 23, no. 7 (2018): 1795, https://doi.org/10.3390/molecules23071795; Gómez-Pinilla, "Brain Foods"; Qingyi Huang et al., "Linking What We Eat"; Kodama et al., "Antioxidant Nutrients"; Larkin et al., "New Risk Factors"; Leonardo C. R. Lima et al., "Consumption of an Anthocyanin-rich Antioxidant Juice Accelerates Recovery of Running Economy and Indirect Markers of Exercise-induced Muscle Damage Following Downhill Running," *Nutrients* 11, no. 10 (2019): 2274, https://doi.org/10.3390/nu11102274; Manivasagam et al., "Role of Oxidative Stress"; Joseph F. Pierre et al., "Dietary Antioxidant Micronutrients Alter Mucosal Inflammatory Risk in a Murine Model of Genetic and Microbial Susceptibility," *The Journal of Nutritional Biochemistry* 54, (2018): 95–104, https://doi.org/10.1016/j.jnutbio.2017.12.002; and Katrin Schütz et al., "Immune-modulating Efficacy of a Polyphenol-rich Beverage on Symptoms Associated with the Common Cold: A Double-blind, Randomised, Placebo-controlled, Multi-Centric Clinical Study," *British Journal of Nutrition* 104, no. 8 (2010): 1156–64, https://doi.org/10.1017/s0007114510002047.

20 Rishikof, *Health Takes Guts.*

21 Akkasheh et al., "Clinical and Metabolic"; Das, Singh, and Nusrat, "Treatment of Asthma"; Ying Guo et al., "Antidepressant Effects of Rosemary Extracts Associate with Anti-inflammatory Effect and Rebalance of Gut Microbiota," *Frontiers in Pharmacology* 9, (2018): 1126, https://doi.org/10.3389/fphar.2018.01126; King et al., "Effectiveness of Probiotics"; Kumperscak et al., "*Lactobacillus Rhamnosus*"; Lang et al., "Nutritional Aspects"; Laursen and Hojsak, "Respiratory Tract Infections"; Lehtoranta, Pitkäranta, and Korpela, "Virus Infections"; Yuying Liu, Jane J. Alookaran, and J. Marc Rhoads, "Probiotics in Autoimmune and Inflammatory Disorders," *Nutrients* 10, no. 10 (2018): 1537, https://doi.org/10.3390/nu10101537; Francois-Pierre J. Martin et al.,"Metabolic Effects of Dark Chocolate Consumption on Energy, Gut Microbiota, and Stress-related Metabolism in Free-living Subjects," *Journal of Proteome Research* 8, no. 12 (2009): 5568–79, https://doi.org/10.1021/pr900607v; Mathee et al., "Gut Microbiome"; Michaël Messaoudi et al., "Assessment of Psychotropic-like Properties of a Probiotic Formulation (Lactobacillus Helveticusr0052 Andbifidobacterium Longumr0175) in Rats and Human Subjects," *British Journal of Nutrition* 105, no. 5 (2010): 755–64, https://doi.org/10.1017/s0007114510004319; Mohammadi et al., "Hypothalamic"; "Probiotics: What You Need to Know," National Center for Complementary and Integrative Health, updated August 2019, https://www.nccih.nih.gov/health/probiotics-what-you-need-to-know; Rishikof, *Health Takes Guts*; Shaaban et al., "The Role of Probiotics"; Takada et al., "Probiotic Lactobacillus Casei"; and Wang et al., "Respiratory Tract Infections."

22 Manas Kotepui, "Diet and Risk of Breast Cancer," *Współczesna Onkologia* 20, no.1 (2016): 13–9, https://doi.org/10.5114/wo.2014.40560; and Mentella et al., "Cancer and Mediterranean Diet."

23 Kassandra L. Munger and Alberto Ascherio, "Prevention and Treatment of MS: Studying the Effects Of Vitamin D," *Multiple Sclerosis Journal* 17, no. 12 (2011): 1405–11, https://doi.org/10.1177/1352458511425366.

24 Haugen and Cook, *Superfood Blender Recipes.*

25 Lauren T. Ptomey et al., "Breakfast Intake and Composition Is Associated with Superior Academic Achievement in Elementary Schoolchildren," *Journal of the American College of Nutrition* 35, no. 4 (2015): 326–33, https://doi.org/10.1080/0731 5724.2015.1048381.

26 Laursen and Hojsak, "Respiratory Tract Infections."

27 Simon Spedding, "Vitamin D and Depression: A Systematic Review and Meta-Analysis Comparing Studies with and without Biological Flaws," *Nutrients* 6, no. 4 (2014): 1501–18, https://doi.org/10.3390/nu6041501.

28 Filipe Lopes Sakamoto et al., "Psychotropic Effects Of L-Theanine and Its Clinical Properties: From the Management of Anxiety and Stress to a Potential Use in Schizophrenia," *Pharmacological Research* 147, (2019): 104395, https://doi.org/10.1016/j.phrs.2019.104395; Ngoc Minh Pham et al., "Green Tea and Coffee Consumption is Inversely Associated with Depressive Symptoms in a Japanese Working Population," *Public Health Nutrition* 17, no. 3 (2013): 625–33, https://doi.org/10.1017/s1368980013000360; Takashi Uebanso et al., "Functional Roles of B-Vitamins in the Gut and Gut Microbiome," *Molecular Nutrition & Food Research* 64, no. 18 (2020): 2000426, https://doi.org/10.1002/mnfr.202000426; and Keiko Unno et al., "Stress-reducing Function of Matcha Green Tea in Animal Experiments and Clinical Trials," *Nutrients* 10, no. 10 (2018): 1468, https://doi.org/10.3390/nu10101468; and ——, "Reduced Stress and Improved Sleep Quality Caused by Green Tea Are Associated with a Reduced Caffeine Content," *Nutrients* 9, no. 7 (2017): 777, https://doi.org/10.3390/nu9070777.

29 Pham et al., "Green Tea."

30 Rishikof, *Health Takes Guts*; Julia J. Rucklidge and Rachel Harrison, "Successful Treatment of Bipolar Disorder II and ADHD with a Micronutrient Formula: A Case Study," *CNS Spectrums* 15, no. 5 (2010): 289–95, https://doi.org/10.1017/s1092852900027516; and Rao Sathyanarayana et al., "Understanding Nutrition, Depression and Mental Illnesses," *Indian Journal of Psychiatry* 50, no. 2 (2008): 77, https://doi.org/10.4103/0019-5545.42391.

31 Kalt et al., "Recent Research"; and Marshall G. Miller et al., "Dietary Blueberry Improves Cognition Among Older Adults in a Randomized, Double-blind, Placebo-controlled Trial," *European Journal of Nutrition* 57, no. 3 (2017): 1169–80, https://doi.org/10.1007/s00394-017-1400-8.

32 Elizabeth J. Johnson et al., "Cognitive Findings of an Exploratory Trial of Docosahexaenoic Acid and Lutein Supplementation in Older Women," *Nutritional Neuroscience* 11, no. 2 (2008): 75–83, https://doi.org/10.1179/147683008x301450.

33 Jeanelle Boyer and Rui Hai Liu, "Apple Phytochemicals and Their Health Benefits," *Nutrition Journal* 3, (2004): 5, https://doi.org/10.1186/1475-2891-3-5.

34 Mentella et al., "Cancer and Mediterranean Diet."

35 Yanyan Li et al., "Sulforaphane, a Dietary Component of Broccoli/Broccoli Sprouts, Inhibits Breast Cancer Stem Cells," *Clinical Cancer Research* 16, no. 9 (2010): 2580–90, https://doi.org/10.1158/1078-0432.ccr-09-2937.

36 Gesch et al., "Influence of Supplementary Vitamins."

37 Ilana Katz Sand, "The Role of Diet in Multiple Sclerosis: Mechanistic Connections and Current Evidence," *Current Nutrition Reports* 7, no. 3 (2018): 150–60, https://doi.org/10.1007/s13668-018-0236-z.

38 Furushima, Ide, and Yamada, "Tea Catechins"; and Shaaban et al., "The Role of Probiotics."

39 Harri Hemilä, "Zinc Lozenges May Shorten the Duration of Colds: A Systematic Review," *The Open Respiratory Medicine Journal* 5, no. 1 (2011): 51–8, https://doi.org/10.2174/1874306401105010051.

40 Appelhans et al., "Depression Severity"; Ines Banjari, Ivana Vukoje, and Milena L. Mandić, "Brain Food: How Nutrition Alters Our Mood and Behavior," *Hrana u Zdravlju i Bolesti, Znanstveno-stručni Časopis za Nutricionizam i Dijetetiku* 3, no.

1 (2014): 13-21, https://www.researchgate.net/publication/263620765_BRAIN_
FOOD_HOW_NUTRITION_ALTERS_OUR_MOOD_AND_BEHAVIOUR;
Bauer and Teixeira, "Inflammation in Psychiatric Disorders"; Castro-Rodriguez
and Garcia-Marcos, "Effects of a Mediterranean Diet"; Eaton, Firth, and Sarris,
"Nutrition and Mental Health"; Gómez-Pinilla, "Brain Foods"; Guilleminault et
al., "Diet and Asthma"; Qingyi Huang et al., "Linking What We Eat"; Lang et al.,
"Nutritional Aspects"; Ye Li et al., "Dietary Patterns"; Lien et al., "Soft Drinks";
Mentella et al., "Cancer and Mediterranean Diet"; Munger and Ascherio, "Prevention
and Treatment"; Chang, "Nutrition & Immune Health"; O'Neil et al., "Diet and
Mental Health"; Opie et al., "Mediterranean Dietary Intervention"; Martha E. Payne
et al., "Fruit, Vegetable, and Antioxidant Intakes Are Lower in Older Adults with
Depression," *Journal of the Academy of Nutrition and Dietetics* 112, no. 12 (2012):
2022–7, https://doi.org/10.1016/j.jand.2012.08.026; Quirk et al., "The Association";
Ríos-Hernández et al., "The Mediterranean Diet"; Rishikof, *Health Takes Guts*;
Saghafian et al., "Fruit and Vegetable"; Wright, "Clinical Nutrition"; and Haugen and
Cook, *Superfood Blender Recipes.*

41 David B. Bellinger, Marci S. DeCaro, and Patricia A. S. Ralston, "Mindfulness,
Anxiety, and High-stakes Mathematics Performance in the Laboratory and
Classroom," *Consciousness and Cognition* 37, (2015): 123–32, https://doi.
org/10.1016/j.concog.2015.09.001; Cherpak, "Mindful Eating"; Danah Henriksen,
Carmen Richardson, and Kyle Shack, "Mindfulness and Creativity: Implications for
Thinking and Learning," *Thinking Skills and Creativity* 37, (2020): 100689, https://
doi.org/10.1016/j.tsc.2020.100689; Shian-Ling Keng, Moria J. Smoski, and Clive
J. Robins, "Effects of Mindfulness on Psychological Health: A Review of Empirical
Studies," *Clinical Psychology Review* 31, no. 6 (2011): 1041–56, https://doi.
org/10.1016/j.cpr.2011.04.006; Lee et al., "Mindfulness-based Intervention"; Mark J.
Sciutto et al., "Effects of a School-based Mindfulness Program for Young Children,"
Journal of Child and Family Studies 30, (2021): 1516–27, https://doi.org/10.1007/
s10826-021-01955-x; Xue, Zhang, and Huang, "ADHD Symptoms"; and Fadel
Zeidan et al., "Mindfulness Meditation Improves Cognition: Evidence of Brief Mental
Training," *Consciousness and Cognition* 19, no. 2 (2010): 597–605, https://doi.
org/10.1016/j.concog.2010.03.014.

42 Bellinger, DeCaro, and Ralston, "Mathematics Performance"; Cherpak, "Mindful
Eating"; Henriksen, Richardson, and Shack, "Mindfulness and Creativity";
Christina F. Chick et al., "A School-based Health and Mindfulness Curriculum
Improves Children's Objectively Measured Sleep," *Sleep* 44, no. 2 (2021): A251–2,
https://doi.org/10.1093/sleep/zsab072.640; Keng, Smoski, and Robins, "Effects of
Mindfulness"; Lee et al., "Mindfulness-based Intervention"; Sciutto et al., "School-
based Mindfulness"; Xue, Zhang, and Huang, "ADHD Symptoms"; and Zeidan et al.,
"Mindfulness Meditation."

43 Yanyan Li et al., "Sulforaphane."

44 Anna L. Boggiss et al., "A Systematic Review of Gratitude Interventions: Effects on
Physical Health and Health Behaviors," *Journal of Psychosomatic Research* 135,
(2020): 110165, https://doi.org/10.1016/j.jpsychores.2020.110165; and Laura S.
Redwine et al., "Pilot Randomized Study of a Gratitude Journaling Intervention on
Heart Rate Variability and Inflammatory Biomarkers in Patients With Stage B Heart
Failure," *Psychosomatic Medicine* 78, no. 6 (2016): 667–76, https://doi.org/10.1097/
psy.0000000000000316.

45 *Merriam-Webster*, s.v., "bronchiectasis (*n.*)," accessed July 26, 2021, https://www. merriam-webster.com/dictionary/bronchiectasis.

46 ——, "foxhole (*n.*)," accessed July 26, 2021, https://www.merriam-webster.com/ dictionary/foxhole.

47 Daryl Densford, "In the Foxhole (a Soldier's Poem)," The Chaplain Kit, March 25, 2016, https://thechaplainkit.com/2016/03/25/in-the-foxhole-a-soldiers-poem/; *Merriam-Webster*, s.v., "foxhole (*n.*)," accessed July 26, 2021, https://www.merriam-webster.com/dictionary/foxhole; and Rachel Synder, "Foxhole Prayers and Why God Is Not Like the Mafia," *ChurchLeaders* (blog), March 20, 2012, https://churchleaders.com/worship/worship-articles/159208-foxhole-prayers-and-why-god-is-not-like-the-mafia.html.

48 Puertollano et al., "Dietary Antioxidants"; Alvarez-Arellano et al., "Potential Target"; Bendich, "Physiological Role"; Iris F. F. Benzie and Sissi Wachtel-Galor, eds., *Herbal Medicine: Biomolecular and Clinical Aspects,* 2nd ed. (Florida: CRC Press, 2011); Sergey A. Fedoreyev et al., "Antiviral and Antioxidant Properties of Echinochrome A," *Marine Drugs* 16, no. 12 (2018): 509, https://doi.org/10.3390/md16120509; Gautam et al., "Role of Antioxidants"; Gesch et al., "Influence of Supplementary Vitamins"; Frank D. Gilliland et al., "Dietary Magnesium, Potassium, Sodium, and Children's Lung Function," *American Journal of Epidemiology* 155, no. 2 (2002): 125–31, https://doi.org/10.1093/aje/155.2.125; Qingyi Huang et al., "Linking What We Eat"; Zhiyi Huang et al., "Role of Vitamin A in the Immune System," *Journal of Clinical Medicine* 7, no. 9 (2018): 258, https://doi.org/10.3390/jcm7090258; Janice K. Kiecolt-Glaser, Heather M. Derry, and Christopher P. Fagundes, "Inflammation: Depression Fans the Flames and Feasts on the Heat," *American Journal of Psychiatry* 172, no. 11 (2015): 1075–91, https://doi.org/10.1176/appi.ajp.2015.15020152; Kodama et al., "Antioxidant Nutrients"; Larkin et al., "New Risk Factors"; Lima et al., "Antioxidant Juice"; Manivasagam et al., "Role of Oxidative Stress"; Mentella et al., "Cancer and Mediterranean Diet"; Moon, *The MIND Diet*; Meri P. Nantz et al., "Consumption of Cranberry Polyphenols Enhances Human-T Cell Proliferation and Reduces the Number of Symptoms Associated with Colds and Influenza: A Randomized, Placebo-controlled Intervention Study," *Nutrition Journal* 12, no. 1 (2013): 161, https://doi.org/10.1186/1475-2891-12-161; Opie et al., "Mediterranean Dietary Intervention"; Payne et al., "Antioxidant Intakes"; Pham et al., "Green Tea"; Ghazal Rahmani et al., "Garlic (*Allium Sativum*) Improves Anxiety- and Depressive-related Behaviors and Brain Oxidative Stress in Diabetic Rats," *Archives of Physiology and Biochemistry* 126, no. 2 (2018): 95–100, https://doi.org/10.1080/13813455.2018. 149474; Rishikof, *Health Takes Guts*; Saghafian et al., "Fruit and Vegetable"; Rossella Sgarbanti et al., "Intracellular Redox State as Target for Anti-Influenza Therapy: Are Antioxidants Always Effective?" *Current Topics in Medicinal Chemistry* 14, no. 22 (2014): 2529–41, https://doi.org/10.2174/1568026614666141203125211; Verlaet et al., "Rationale"; and Haugen and Cook, *Superfood Blender Recipes.*

49 Rishikof, *Health Takes Guts*; and Deledda et al., "Diet-derived Antioxidants."

50 Puertollano et al., "Dietary Antioxidants"; Bendich, "Physiological Role"; Furushima, Ide, and Yamada, "Tea Catechins"; Morgan R. Griffin, "Natural Cold and Flu Remedies: Americans Are Turning to Cold and Flu Supplements in Greater Numbers," *WebMD*, reviewed December 29, 2010, https://www.webmd.com/a-to-z-guides/ features/colds-flu-immune-system#1; Guillin et al., "Selenium"; Harri Hemilä, "Vitamin C and Community-acquired Pneumonia," *American Journal of Respiratory and Critical Care Medicine* 184, no. 5 (2011): 621–2, https://doi.org/10.1164/

ajrccm.184.5.621a; ——, "Vitamin C and Infections," *Nutrients* 9, no. 4 (2017): 339, https://doi.org/10.3390/nu9040339; Zhiyi Huang et al., "Role of Vitamin A"; Klemm, "Support"; J. Rodrigo Mora, Makoto Iwata, and Ulrich H. von Andrian, "Vitamin Effects on the Immune System: Vitamins A and D Take Centre Stage," *Nature Reviews Immunology* 8, no. 9 (2008): 685–98, https://doi.org/10.1038/nri2378; Nantz et al., "Cranberry Polyphenols"; David C. Nieman et al., "Quercetin Reduces Illness but Not Immune Perturbations after Intensive Exercise," *Medicine & Science in Sports & Exercise* 39, no. 9 (2007): 1561–9, https://doi.org/10.1249/mss.0b013e318076b566; Chang, "Nutrition & Immune Health"; Rishikof, *Health Takes Guts*; Sgarbanti et al., "Intracellular Redox State"; Somerville, Braakhuis, and Hopkins, "Effect of Flavonoids"; and Haugen and Cook, *Superfood Blender Recipes*.

51 Puertollano et al., "Dietary Antioxidants"; Alvarez-Arellano et al., "Potential Target"; Bendich, "Physiological Role"; Benzie and Wachtel-Galor, *Herbal Medicine*"; Sergey A. Fedoreyev et al., "Antiviral and Antioxidant Properties of Echinochrome A," *Marine Drugs* 16, no. 12 (2018): 509, https://doi.org/10.3390/md16120509; Gautam et al., "Role of Antioxidants"; Gesch et al., "Influence of Supplementary Vitamins"; Gilliland et al., "Children's Lung Function"; Qingyi Huang et al., "Linking What We Eat"; Zhiyi Huang et al., "Role of Vitamin A in the Immune System," *Journal of Clinical Medicine* 7, no. 9 (2018): 258, https://doi.org/10.3390/jcm7090258; Janice K. Kiecolt-Glaser, Heather M. Derry, and Christopher P. Fagundes, "Inflammation: Depression Fans the Flames and Feasts on the Heat," *American Journal of Psychiatry* 172, no. 11 (2015): 1075–91, https://doi.org/10.1176/appi.ajp.2015.15020152; Kodama et al., "Antioxidant Nutrients"; Larkin et al., "New Risk Factors"; Lima et al., "Antioxidant Juice"; Manivasagam et al., "Role of Oxidative Stress"; Mentella et al., "Cancer and Mediterranean Diet"; Moon, *The MIND Diet*; Meri P. Nantz et al., "Consumption of Cranberry Polyphenols Enhances Human-T Cell Proliferation and Reduces the Number of Symptoms Associated with Colds and Influenza: A Randomized, Placebo-controlled Intervention Study," *Nutrition Journal* 12, no. 1 (2013): 161, https://doi.org/10.1186/1475-2891-12-161; Opie et al., "Mediterranean Dietary Intervention"; Payne et al., "Antioxidant Intakes"; Pham et al., "Green Tea"; Ghazal Rahmani et al., "Garlic (*Allium Sativum*) Improves Anxiety- and Depressive-related Behaviors and Brain Oxidative Stress in Diabetic Rats," *Archives of Physiology and Biochemistry* 126, no. 2 (2018): 95–100, https://doi.org/10.1080/13813455.2018. 149474; Rishikof, *Health Takes Guts*; Saghafian et al., "Fruit and Vegetable"; Rossella Sgarbanti et al., "Intracellular Redox State as Target for Anti-Influenza Therapy: Are Antioxidants Always Effective?" *Current Topics in Medicinal Chemistry* 14, no. 22 (2014): 2529–41, https://doi.org/10.2174/1568026614666141203125211; Verlaet et al., "Rationale"; and Haugen and Cook, *Superfood Blender Recipes*.

52 Bauer and Teixeira, "Inflammation in Psychiatric Disorders"; Wright, "Beyond Food and Mood"; Gautam et al., "Role of Antioxidants"; Qingyi Huang et al., "Linking What We Eat"; Felice N. Jacka, "Nutritional Psychiatry: Where to Next?" *EBioMedicine* 17, (2017): 24–9, https://doi.org/10.1016/j.ebiom.2017.02.020; —— et al., "Controlled Trial"; Khalid et al., "Blueberry Flavonoids"; Kiecolt-Glaser, Derry, and Fagundes, "Inflammation"; Lang et al., "Nutritional Aspects"; Ye Li et al., "Dietary Patterns"; Magalhães et al., "Antioxidant Treatments"; O'Neil et al., "Diet and Mental Health"; Opie et al., "Mediterranean Dietary Intervention"; Payne et al., "Antioxidant Intakes"; Pham et al., "Green Tea"; Quirk et al., "The Association"; Rishikof, *Health Takes Guts*; Saghafian et al., "Fruit and Vegetable"; Salim, Chugh, and Asghar, "Inflammation in Anxiety"; Sarris et al., "Nutritional Medicine";

Schneiderman, Ironson, and Siegel, "Stress and Health"; and Haugen and Cook, *Superfood Blender Recipes.*

53 Kotepui, "Breast Cancer"; Moon, *The MIND Diet*; Rishikof, *Health Takes Guts*; and Haugen and Cook, *Superfood Blender Recipes.*

54 Kalt et al., "Recent Research"; Moon, *The MIND Diet*; Rishikof, *Health Takes Guts*; and Haugen and Cook, *Superfood Blender Recipes.*

55 Rishikof, *Health Takes Guts*; and Haugen and Cook, *Superfood Blender Recipes.*

56 Gómez-Pinilla, "Brain Foods"; Kalt et al., "Recent Research"; Miller et al., "Dietary Blueberry"; Moon, *The MIND Diet*; and Schütz et al., "Immune-modulating Efficacy."

57 Alyssa Salz, "Substance Abuse and Nutrition," *Today's Dietitian* 16, no. 12 (2014): 44, https://www.todaysdietitian.com/newarchives/120914p44.shtml; and Haugen and Cook, *Superfood Blender Recipes.*

58 Alvarez-Arellano et al., "Potential Target"; Hewedi, Mostafa, and El Hadidi, "Egyptian Children"; Manivasagam et al., "Role of Oxidative Stress"; Ríos-Hernández et al., "The Mediterranean Diet"; Rishikof, Health Takes Guts; Verlaet et al., "Rationale"; and Wendy Weber and Sanford Newmark, "Complementary and Alternative Medical Therapies for Attention-Deficit/Hyperactivity Disorder and Autism," *Pediatric Clinics of North America* 54, no. 6 (2007): 983–1006, https://doi.org/10.1016/j.pcl.2007.09.006.

59 Ya-Jie Bai and Ru-Jun Dai, "Serum Levels of Vitamin A and 25-Hydroxyvitamin D3 (25OHD3) as Reflectors of Pulmonary Function and Quality of Life (QOL) in Children with Stable Asthma," *Medicine* 97, no. 7 (2018): e9830, https://doi.org/10.1097/md.0000000000009830; Boyer and Liu, "Apple Phytochemicals"; Castro-Rodriguez and Garcia-Marcos, "Effects of a Mediterranean Diet"; Guilleminault et al., "Diet and Asthma"; Kodama et al., "Antioxidant Nutrients"; Larkin et al., "New Risk Factors"; and Rishikof, *Health Takes Guts.*

60 Brambilla et al., "Role of Antioxidant Supplement"; Kalt et al., "Recent Research"; Sand, "Multiple Sclerosis"; and Rishikof, *Health Takes Guts.*

61 Cerhan et al., "Antioxidant Micronutrients"; and Rishikof, *Health Takes Guts.*

62 Kalt et al., "Recent Research"; and Yanyan Li et al., "Sulforaphane."

63 Boyer and Liu, "Apple Phytochemicals."

64 Goutam Brahmachari, ed., *Discovery and Development of Anti-Inflammatory Agents from Natural Products*, 1st ed., vol. 4 of *Natural Product Drug Discovery* (Amsterdam: Elsevier, 2019).

65 Karen Mumme and Welma Stonehouse, "Effects of Medium-Chain Triglycerides on Weight Loss and Body Composition: A Meta-Analysis of Randomized Controlled Trials," *Journal of the Academy of Nutrition and Dietetics* 115, no. 2 (2015): 249–63, https://doi.org/10.1016/j.jand.2014.10.022; Densie Webb, "Herbs and Spices: Holiday Spices," *Today's Dietitian* 18, no. 11 (November 2016): 14, https://www.todaysdietitian.com/newarchives/1116p14.shtml; and Dimas Rahadian Aji Muhammad and Koen Dewettinck, "Cinnamon and Its Derivatives as Potential Ingredient in Functional Food—A Review," *International Journal of Food Properties* 20, sup. 2 (2017): 2237–63, https://doi.org/10.1080/10942912.2017.1369102.

66 Rishikof, *Health Takes Guts*; and A. P. Simopoulos, "The Importance of the Ratio of Omega-6/Omega-3 Essential Fatty Acids," *Biomedicine & Pharmacotherapy* 56, no. 8 (2002): 365–79, https://doi.org/10.1016/s0753-3322(02)00253-6.

67 Banjari, Vukoje, and Mandić, "Brain Food"; Eaton, Firth, and Sarris, "Nutrition and Mental Health"; Qingyi Huang et al., "Linking What We Eat"; Jacka,

"Nutritional Psychiatry"; Lang et al., "Nutritional Aspects"; Anne Berit C. Samuelsen, Jürgen Schrezenmeir, and Svein H. Knutsen, "Effects of Orally Administered Yeast-Derived Beta-Glucans: A Review," *Molecular Nutrition & Food Research* 58, no. 1 (2013): 183–93, https://doi.org/10.1002/mnfr.201300338; and Wright, "Beyond Food and Mood."

68 Amelia R. Sherry, "Vitamin B12," *Today's Dietitian* 16, no 8 (2014): 20, https://www.todaysdietitian.com/newarchives/080114p20.shtml.

69 Christine Tara Peterson et al., "B Vitamins and Their Role in Immune Regulation and Cancer," *Nutrients* 12, no. 11 (2020): 3380, https://doi.org/10.3390/nu12113380; "Foods High in B Vitamins," Diet & Weight Management, Nourish by WebMD, reviewed on December 13, 2020, https://www.webmd.com/diet/foods-high-in-b-vitamins#1; and Haugen and Cook, *Superfood Blender Recipes.*

70 Peterson et al., "Immune Regulation"; Uebanso et al., "Gut Microbiome"; and Haugen and Cook, *Superfood Blender Recipes.*

71 Salz, "Substance Abuse"; and Haugen and Cook, *Superfood Blender Recipes.*

72 Sherry, "Vitamin B12."

73 Kiah Bertoglio et al., "Pilot Study of the Effect of Methyl B12 Treatment on Behavioral and Biomarker Measures in Children with Autism," *The Journal of Alternative and Complementary Medicine* 16, no. 5 (2010a): 555–60, https://doi.org/10.1089/acm.2009.0177; S. Jill James et al., "Efficacy of Methylcobalamin and Folinic Acid Treatment on Glutathione Redox Status in Children with Autism," *The American Journal of Clinical Nutrition* 89, no. 1 (2008): 425–30, https://doi.org/10.3945/ajcn.2008.26615; and M. Mousain-Bosc et al., "Improvement of Neurobehavioral Disorders in Children Supplemented with Magnesium-Vitamin B6. I. Attention Deficit Hyperactivity Disorders," *Magnesium Research* 19, no. 1 (2006): 46–52, https://pubmed.ncbi.nlm.nih.gov/16846100/.

74 "Potassium," National Institutes of Health, accessed July 27, 2021, https://ods.od.nih.gov/factsheets/Potassium-HealthProfessional/.

75 Michael H. Bloch and Ahmad Qawasmi, "Omega-3 Fatty Acid Supplementation for the Treatment of Children With Attention-deficit/Hyperactivity Disorder Symptomatology: Systematic Review and Meta-Analysis," *Journal of the American Academy of Child and Adolescent Psychiatry* 50, no. 10, (2011): 991–1000, https://doi.org/10.1016/j.jaac.2011.06.008; Lang et al., "Nutritional Aspects"; and Mikirova et al., "Metabolic Correction."

76 Griffin, "Natural Cold"; Hemilä, "Zinc Lozenges"; Klemm, "Support"; Mariangela Rondanelli et al., "Self-care for Common Colds: The Pivotal Role of Vitamin D, Vitamin C, Zinc, and *Echinacea* in Three Main Immune Interactive Clusters (Physical Barriers, Innate and Adaptive Immunity) Involved during an Episode of Common Colds—Practical Advice on Dosages and on the Time to Take These Nutrients/Botanicals in order to Prevent or Treat Common Colds," *Evidence-Based Complementary and Alternative Medicine* 2018, (2018): 1–36, https://doi.org/10.1155/2018/5813095; A. H. Shankar and A. S. Prasad, "Zinc and Immune Function: The Biological Basis of Altered Resistance to Infection," *The American Journal of Clinical Nutrition* 68, no. 2 (1998): 447S–63S, https://doi.org/10.1093/ajcn/68.2.447s; and Meenu Singh and Rashmi R. Das, "Zinc for the Common Cold," *Cochrane Database of Systematic Reviews*, no. 6 (2013): CD001364, https://doi.org/10.1002/14651858.cd001364.pub4.

77 Rishikof, *Health Takes Guts*; and Salz, "Substance Abuse."

78 Health Information, "Iron," Office of Dietary Supplements, National Institutes of Health, accessed July 31, 2021, https://ods.od.nih.gov/factsheets/Iron-Consumer/; and Haugen and Cook, *Superfood Blender Recipes.*

79 "Iron," National Institutes of Health.

80 "Magnesium," Office of Dietary Supplements, National Institutes of Health, accessed July 31, 2021, https://ods.od.nih.gov/factsheets/Magnesium-Consumer/; and Haugen and Cook, *Superfood Blender Recipes.*

81 Gilliland et al., "Children's Lung Function"; Lang et al., "Nutritional Aspects"; "Magnesium," National Institutes of Health and Wright, "Beyond Food and Mood."

82 "Magnesium," National Institutes of Health.

83 "Calcium," Office of Dietary Supplements, National Institutes of Health, accessed July 31, 2021, https://ods.od.nih.gov/factsheets/Calcium-HealthProfessional/; and Haugen and Cook, *Superfood Blender Recipes.*

84 Makki et al., "Dietary Fiber"; and Haugen and Cook, *Superfood Blender Recipes.*

85 Kotepui, "Breast Cancer"; and Yang Yang et al., "All-Cause Mortality."

86 Mohammed Iddir et al., "Strengthening the Immune System and Reducing Inflammation and Oxidative Stress through Diet and Nutrition: Considerations During the COVID-19 Crisis," *Nutrients* 12, no. 6 (2020): 1562, https://doi.org/10.3390/nu12061562.

87 Rishikof, *Health Takes Guts*; Yang Yang et al., "All-Cause Mortality"; and Haugen and Cook, *Superfood Blender Recipes.*

88 Yang Yang et al., "All-Cause Mortality."

89 Anna K. E. Vadell et al., "Anti-inflammatory Diet in Rheumatoid Arthritis (ADIRA)—A Randomized, Controlled Crossover Trial Indicating Effects on Disease Activity," *The American Journal of Clinical Nutrition* 111, no. 6 (2020): 1203–13, https://doi.org/10.1093/ajcn/nqaa019.

90 Yang Yang et al., "All-Cause Mortality"; and Haugen and Cook, *Superfood Blender Recipes.*

91 Haugen and Cook, *Superfood Blender Recipes.*

92 Miki et al., "Japanese Employees."

93 Yang Yang et al., "All-Cause Mortality"; and Haugen and Cook, *Superfood Blender Recipes.*

94 John Jacob Cannell, "Vitamin D and Autism, What's New?" *Reviews in Endocrine and Metabolic Disorders* 18, no. 2 (2017): 183–93, https://doi.org/10.1007/s11154-017-9409-0; Gómez-Pinilla, "Brain Foods"; Hansen et al., "Forensic Inpatients"; Lauren R. Harms et al., "Vitamin D and the Brain," *Best Practice & Research Clinical Endocrinology & Metabolism* 25, no. 4 (2011): 657–69, https://doi.org/10.1016/j.beem.2011.05.009; Qingyi Huang et al., "Linking What We Eat"; Jacka, "Nutritional Psychiatry"; David A. Jolliffe et al., "Vitamin D Supplementation to Prevent Asthma Exacerbations: A Systematic Review and Meta-Analysis of Individual Participant Data," *The Lancet Respiratory Medicine* 5, no. 11 (2017): 881–90, https://doi.org/10.1016/s2213-2600(17)30306-5; Kotepui, "Breast Cancer"; Lang et al., "Nutritional Aspects"; "Low Vitamin D Levels Associated with Colds and Flu," NIH Research Matters, National Institutes of Health, posted April 4, 2016, https://www.nih.gov/news-events/nih-research-matters/low-vitamin-d-levels-associated-colds-flu; Mora, Iwata, and von Andrian, "Centre Stage"; Rishikof, *Health Takes Guts*; Rondanelli et al., "Self-care"; and Spedding, "Biological Flaws."

95 "Vitamin K," Office of Dietary Supplements, National Institutes of Health, accessed July 31, 2021, https://ods.od.nih.gov/factsheets/vitamink-consumer/.

96 Rishikof, *Health Takes Guts*; and Vadell et al., "Disease Activity."

97 Joseph Charles Maroon and Jeffrey W. Bost, "Omega-3 Fatty Acids (Fish Oil) as an Anti-inflammatory: An Alternative to Nonsteroidal Anti-inflammatory Drugs for Discogenic Pain," *Surgical Neurology* 65, no. 4 (2006): 326–31, https://doi.org/10.1016/j.surneu.2005.10.023; and Rishikof, *Health Takes Guts*.

98 Boyer and Liu, "Apple Phytochemicals"; Fernandes, Mutch, and Leri, "Brain Regions"; Fristad et al., "Psychoeducational Psychotherapy"; Hansen et al., "Forensic Inpatients"; Qingyi Huang et al., "Linking What We Eat"; Jacka, "Nutritional Psychiatry"; Lang et al., "Nutritional Aspects"; Ye Li et al., "Dietary Patterns"; Su, Matsuoka, and Pae, "Prevention of Mood"; Wright, "Beyond Food and Mood"; and Andrea S. Young et al., "Psychoeducational Psychotherapy and Omega-3 Supplementation Improve Co-Occurring Behavioral Problems in Youth with Depression: Results from a Pilot RCT," *Journal of Abnormal Child Psychology* 45, no. 5 (2016): 1025–37, https://doi.org/10.1007/s10802-016-0203-3.

99 "Monounsaturated Fat," American Heart Association, last reviewed June 1, 2015, accessed July 31, 2021, https://www.heart.org/en/healthy-living/healthy-eating/eat-smart/fats/monounsaturated-fats.

100 Rishikof, *Health Takes Guts*.

101 Gómez-Pinilla, "Brain Foods"; and Moon, *The MIND Diet*.

102 Gómez-Pinilla, "Brain Foods"; and Moon, *The MIND Diet*.

103 Salz, "Substance Abuse"; and Haugen and Cook, *Superfood Blender Recipes*.

104 Adams et al., "Asthma Endpoints"; Jun Miyata and Makoto Arita, "Role of Omega-3 Fatty Acids and Their Metabolites in Asthma and Allergic Diseases," *Allergology International* 64, no. 1 (2015): 27–34, https://doi.org/10.1016/j.alit.2014.08.003; and Stoodley et al., "Higher Omega-3 Index."

105 Abdullah et al., "Reducing ADHD"; J. G. Bell et al., "Essential Fatty Acids and Phospholipase A2 in Autistic Spectrum Disorders," *Prostaglandins, Leukotrienes and Essential Fatty Acids* 71, no. 4 (2004): 201–4, https://doi.org/10.1016/j.plefa.2004.03.008; Michael H. Bloch and Jilian Mulqueen, "Nutritional Supplements for the Treatment of ADHD," *Child and Adolescent Psychiatric Clinics of North America* 23, no. 4 (2014): 883–97, https://doi.org/10.1016/j.chc.2014.05.002; Bloch and Qawasmi, "Attention-deficit/Hyperactivity Disorder"; Cooper et al., "Emotional Dysregulation"; Stewart M. Johnson and Eric Hollander, "Evidence That Eicosapentaenoic Acid is Effective in Treating Autism," *The Journal of Clinical Psychiatry* 64, no. 7 (2003): 848–9, https://doi.org/10.4088/jcp.v64n0718c; Nagwa A. Meguid et al., "Role of Polyunsaturated Fatty Acids in the Management of Egyptian Children with Autism," *Clinical Biochemistry* 41, no. 13 (2008): 1044–8, https://doi.org/10.1016/j.clinbiochem.2008.05.013; Mikirova et al., "Metabolic Correction"; Milte et al., "Eicosapentaenoic"; and Natalie Sinn and Janet Bryan, "Effect of Supplementation with Polyunsaturated Fatty Acids and Micronutrients on Learning and Behavior Problems Associated with Child ADHD," *Journal of Developmental & Behavioral Pediatrics* 28, no. 2 (2007): 82–91, https://doi.org/10.1097/01.dbp.0000267558.88457.a5.

106 "Monounsaturated Fat," National Institutes of Health.

107 "Probiotics," National Center for Complementary and Integrative Health. and Rishikof, *Health Takes Guts*.

108 Abt et al., "Commensal Bacteria"; Kanauchi et al., "Probiotics and Paraprobiotics"; Kang et al., "Common Cold"; Sarah King et al., "Effectiveness of Probiotics on the Duration of Illness in Healthy Children and Adults Who Develop Common

Acute Respiratory Infectious Conditions: A Systematic Review and Meta-Analysis,"
British Journal of Nutrition 112, no. 1 (2014): 41–54, https://doi.org/10.1017/
s0007114514000075; Laursen and Hojsak, "Respiratory Tract Infections"; Lehtoranta,
Pitkäranta, and Korpela, "Virus Infections"; "Probiotics," National Center for
Complementary and Integrative Health. Rishikof, *Health Takes Guts*; and Wang et al.,
"Respiratory Tract Infections."
109 Brahmachari, *Discovery and Development*; Liu, Alookaran, and Rhoads,
"Probiotics"; Julio Plaza-Díaz et al., "Evidence of the Anti-Inflammatory Effects of
Probiotics and Synbiotics in Intestinal Chronic Diseases," *Nutrients* 9, no. 6 (2017):
555, https://doi.org/10.3390/nu9060555; and Rishikof, *Health Takes Guts*.
110 Akkasheh et al., "Clinical and Metabolic"; Bested, Logan, and Selhub, "Intestinal
Microbiota"; Huang, Wang, and Hu, "Probiotics on Depression"; Jacka,
"Nutritional Psychiatry"; Messaoudi et al., "Psychotropic-like Properties"; —,
"Probiotic Formulation"; Mohammadi et al., "Hypothalamic"; Pärtty et al.,
"Probiotic Intervention"; Rishikof, *Health Takes Guts*; and Takada et al., "Probiotic
Lactobacillus Casei."
111 Rishikof, *Health Takes Guts*; and Haugen and Cook, *Superfood Blender Recipes*.
112 Rishikof, *Health Takes Guts*; and Ram Mohan Thushara et al., "Cardiovascular
Benefits of Probiotics: A Review of Experimental and Clinical Studies," *Food &
Function* 7, no. 2 (2016): 632–42, https://doi.org/10.1039/c5fo01190f.
113 Gesch et al., "Influence of Supplementary Vitamins"; and Pouya Nematolahi
et al., "Effects of Rosmarinus Officinalis L. on Memory Performance, Anxiety,
Depression, and Sleep Quality in University Students: A Randomized Clinical
Trial," *Complementary Therapies in Clinical Practice* 30, (2018): 24–8, https://doi.
org/10.1016/j.ctcp.2017.11.004.
114 Johnson et al., "Cognitive Findings"; Mikirova et al., "Metabolic Correction"; Quirk
et al., "The Association"; and Rishikof, *Health Takes Guts*.
115 Rishikof, *Health Takes Guts*; and Haugen and Cook, *Superfood Blender Recipes*.
116 Das, Singh, and Nusrat, "Treatment of Asthma"; Yusuf Nazir et al., "Probiotics and
Their Potential Preventive and Therapeutic Role for Cancer, High Serum Cholesterol,
and Allergic and HIV Diseases," *BioMed Research International* 2018, ID 3428437
(2018): 1–17, https://doi.org/10.1155/2018/3428437; "Probiotics," National Center
for Complementary and Integrative Health and G. Vighi et al., "Allergy and the
Gastrointestinal System," *Clinical & Experimental Immunology* 153, suppl. 1 (2008):
3–6, https://doi.org/10.1111/j.1365-2249.2008.03713.x.
117 Bull-Larsen and Mohajeri, "Bacterial Microbiome"; Sand, "Multiple Sclerosis";
Kumperscak et al., "*Lactobacillus Rhamnosus*"; Ng et al., "Autism Spectrum
Disorders"; and Shaaban et al., "The Role of Probiotics."
118 Diet & Weight Management, "B Vitamins"; Wright, "Beyond Food and Mood";
and Zizhen Xie et al., "A Review of Sleep Disorders and Melatonin," *Neurological
Research* 39, no. 6 (2017): 559–65, https://doi.org/10.1080/01616412.2017.1315864.
119 Shinsuke Hidese et al., "Effects of L-Theanine Administration on Stress-Related
Symptoms and Cognitive Functions in Healthy Adults: A Randomized Controlled
Trial," *Nutrients* 11, no. 10 (2019): 2362, https://doi.org/10.3390/nu11102362;
Sakamoto et al., "Psychotropic Effects"; Unno et al., "Stress-reducing Function"; and
—, "Anti-stress Effects of Drinking Green Tea with Lowered Caffeine and Enriched
Theanine, Epigallocatechin and Arginine on Psychosocial Stress Induced Adrenal
Hypertrophy in Mice," *Phytomedicine*, 23, no. 12 (2016): 1365–74, https://doi.
org/10.1016/j.phymed.2016.07.006.

228   LACY NGO

120 A. Juszkiewicz et al., "The Effect of L-Theanine Supplementation on the Immune System of Athletes Exposed to Strenuous Physical Exercise," *Journal of the International Society of Sports Nutrition* 16, no. 1 (2019): 7, https://doi.org/10.1186/s12970-019-0274-y.

121 Samuelsen, Schrezenmeir, and Knutsen, "Beta-Glucans."

122 "Beta-Glucans: Uses, Side Effects, and More" Overview, WebMD accessed July 31, 2021, https://www.webmd.com/vitamins/ai/ingredientmono-1041/beta-glucans.

123 Glyn Howatson et al., "Effect of Tart Cherry Juice (Prunus Cerasus) on Melatonin Levels and Enhanced Sleep Quality," *European Journal of Nutrition* 51, no. 8 (2011): 909–16, https://doi.org/10.1007/s00394-011-0263-7; and Xie et al., "Melatonin."

124 Luciana Besedovsky, Tanja Lange, and Jan Born, "Sleep and Immune Function," *Pflügers Archiv - European Journal of Physiology* 463, no. 1 (2011): 121–37, https://doi.org/10.1007/s00424-011-1044-0; Michael J. Peterson and Ruth M. Benca, "Sleep in Mood Disorders," *Psychiatric Clinics of North America* 29, no. 4 (2006): 1009–32, https://doi.org/10.1016/j.psc.2006.09.003; Meredith E. Rumble, Kaitlin Hanley White, and Ruth M. Benca, "Sleep Disturbances in Mood Disorders," *Psychiatric Clinics of North America* 38, no. 4 (2015): 743–59, https://doi.org/10.1016/j.psc.2015.07.006; and Alexei Verkhratsky et al., "Editorial: Sleep and Mood Disorders," *Frontiers in Psychiatry* 10, (2020): 981, https://doi.org/10.3389/fpsyt.2019.00981.

125 Castro-Rodriguez and Garcia-Marcos, "Effects of a Mediterranean Diet"; Shao-Min Chang and Chung-Hey Chen, "Effects of an Intervention with Drinking Chamomile Tea on Sleep Quality and Depression in Sleep Disturbed Postnatal Women: A Randomized Controlled Trial," *Journal of Advanced Nursing* 72, no. 2 (2016): 306–15, https://doi.org/10.1111/jan.12836; Lehtoranta, Pitkäranta, and Korpela, "Virus Infections"; and Jun J. Mao et al., "Long-term Chamomile (Matricaria Chamomilla L.) Treatment for Generalized Anxiety Disorder: A Randomized Clinical Trial," *Phytomedicine* 23, no. 14 (2016): 1735–42, https://doi.org/10.1016/j.phymed.2016.10.012.

126 Chang and Chen, "Chamomile Tea," 306–315.

127 Appelhans et al., "Depression Severity"; Banjari, Vukoje, and Mandić, "Brain Food"; Bauer and Teixeira, "Inflammation in Psychiatric Disorders"; Castro-Rodriguez and Garcia-Marcos, "Effects of a Mediterranean Diet"; Wright, "Beyond Food and Mood"; Eaton, Firth, and Sarris, "Nutrition and Mental Health"; Gómez-Pinilla, "Brain Foods"; Guilleminault et al., "Diet and Asthma"; Qingyi Huang et al., "Linking What We Eat"; Lang et al., "Nutritional Aspects"; Ye Li et al., "Dietary Patterns"; Lien et al., "Soft Drinks"; Mentella et al., "Cancer and Mediterranean Diet"; Munger and Ascherio, "Prevention and Treatment"; Chang, "Nutrition & Immune Health"; O'Neil et al., "Diet and Mental Health"; Opie et al., "Mediterranean Dietary Intervention"; Payne et al., "Antioxidant Intakes"; Quirk et al., "The Association"; Ríos-Hernández et al., "The Mediterranean Diet"; Rishikof, *Health Takes Guts*; Saghafian et al., "Fruit and Vegetable"; and Haugen and Cook, *Superfood Blender Recipes*.

128 ——.

129 C. Perrier and B. Corthésy, "Gut Permeability and Food Allergies," *Clinical & Experimental Allergy* 41, no. 1 (2010): 20–8, https://doi.org/10.1111/j.1365-2222.2010.03639.x; Rishikof, *Health Takes Guts*; and William Zhao, His-En Ho, and Supinda Bunyavanich, "The Gut Microbiome in Food Allergy," *Annals of Allergy, Asthma & Immunology* 122, no. 3 (2019): 276–82, https://doi.org/10.1016/j.anai.2018.12.012.

130 Donna McCann et al., "Food Additives and Hyperactive Behaviour in 3-Year-Old and 8/9-Year-Old Children in the Community: A Randomised, Double-blinded, Placebo-controlled Trial," *Lancet* 370, no. 9598 (2007): 1560–7, https://doi.org/10.1016/s0140-6736(07)61306-3; and Lidy M. Pelsser et al., "Effects of a Restricted Elimination Diet on the Behaviour of Children with Attention-Deficit Hyperactivity Disorder (INCA Study): A Randomised Controlled Trial," *Lancet* 377, no. 9764 (2011): 494–503, https://doi.org/10.1016/s0140-6736(10)62227-1.

BIBLIOGRAPHY

"Food Guidelines." Blue Zones. September 7, 2020. https://www.bluezones.com/recipes/food-guidelines/.

Abdullah, Muhammad, Benjamin Jowett, Paula Jane Whittaker, and Lesley Patterson. "The Effectiveness of Omega-3 Supplementation in Reducing ADHD Associated Symptoms in Children as Measured by the Conners' Rating Scales: A Systematic Review of Randomized Controlled Trials." *Journal of Psychiatric Research* 110 (2019): 64–73. https://doi.org/10.1016/j.jpsychires.2018.12.002.

Abt, Michael C., Lisa C. Osborne, Laurel A. Monticelli, Travis A. Doering, Theresa Alenghat, Gregory F. Sonnenberg, Micheal A. Paley, Marcelo Antenus, Katie L. Williams, Jan Erikson, E. John Wherry, and David Artis. "Commensal Bacteria Calibrate the Activation Threshold of Innate Antiviral Immunity." *Immunity* 37, no. 1 (2012): 158–70. https://doi.org/10.1016/j.immuni.2012.04.011.

Adams, Shahieda, Andreas L. Lopata, Cornelius M. Smuts, Roslynn Baatjies, and Mohamed F. Jeebhay. "Relationship Between Serum Omega-3 Fatty Acid and Asthma Endpoints." *International Journal of Environmental Research and Public Health* 16, no. 1 (2018): 43. https://doi.org/10.3390/ijerph16010043.

Akkasheh, Ghodarz, Zahra Kashani-Poor, Maryam Tajabadi-Ebrahimi, Parvaneh Jafari, Hossein Akbari, Mohsen Taghizadeh, Mohammad Reza Memarzadeh, Zatollah Asemi, and Ahmad Esmaillzadeh. "Clinical and Metabolic Response to Probiotic Administration in Patients with Major Depressive Disorder: A Randomized, Double-blind, Placebo-controlled Trial." *Nutrition* 32, no. 3 (2016): 315–20. https://doi.org/10.1016/j.nut.2015.09.003.

Alvarez-Arellano, Lourdes, Nadia González-García, Marcela Salazar-García, and Juan Carlos Corona. "Antioxidants as a Potential Target Against Inflammation and Oxidative Stress in Attention-deficit/Hyperactivity Disorder." *Antioxidants* 9, no. 2 (2020): 176. https://doi.org/10.3390/antiox9020176.

American Heart Association.. "Monounsaturated Fat." Last reviewed June 1, 2015. Accesssed July 31, 2021. https://www.heart.org/en/healthy-living/healthy-eating/eat-smart/fats/monounsaturated-fats.

Appelhans, Bradley M., Matthew C. Whited, Kristin L. Schneider, Yunsheng Ma, Jesica L. Oleski, Philip A. Merriam, Molly E. Waring, Barbara C. Olendzki, Devin M. Mann, Ira S. Ockene, and Sherry L. Pagoto. "Depression Severity, Diet Quality, and Physical Activity in Women with Obesity and Depression." *Journal of the Academy of Nutrition and Dietetics* 112, no. 5 (2012): 693–8. https://doi.org/10.1016/j.jand.2012.02.006.

Aust, J., and T. Bradshaw. "Mindfulness Interventions for Psychosis: A Systematic Review of the Literature." *Journal of Psychiatric and Mental Health Nursing* 24, no. 1 (2016): 69–83. https://doi.org/10.1111/jpm.12357.

Bai, Ya-Jie, and Ru-Jun Dai. "Serum Levels of Vitamin A and 25-Hydroxyvitamin D3 (25OHD3) as Reflectors of Pulmonary Function and Quality of Life (QOL) in Children with Stable Asthma." *Medicine* 97, no. 7 (2018): e9830. https://doi.org/10.1097/md.0000000000009830.

Banjari, Ines, Ivana Vukoje, and Milena L. Mandić. "Brain Food: How Nutrition Alters Our Mood and Behavior." *Hrana u Zdravlju i Bolesti, Znanstveno-stručni Časopis za Nutricionizam i Dijetetiku* 3, no. 1 (2014): 13-21. https://www.researchgate.net/publication/263620765_BRAIN_FOOD_HOW_NUTRITION_ALTERS_OUR_MOOD_AND_BEHAVIOUR.

Bauer, Moisés E., and Antonio L. Teixeira. "Inflammation in Psychiatric Disorders: What Comes First?" *Annals of the New York Academy of Sciences* 1437, no. 1 (2018): 57–67. https://doi.org/10.1111/nyas.13712.

Bell, J. G., E. E. MacKinlay, J. R. Dick, D. J. MacDonald, R. M. Boyle, and A. C. A. Glen. "Essential Fatty Acids and Phospholipase A2 in Autistic Spectrum Disorders." *Prostaglandins, Leukotrienes and Essential Fatty Acids* 71, no. 4 (2004): 201–4. https://doi.org/10.1016/j.plefa.2004.03.008.

Bellinger, David B., Marci S. DeCaro, and Patricia A. S. Ralston. "Mindfulness, Anxiety, and High-stakes Mathematics Performance in the Laboratory and Classroom." *Consciousness and Cognition* 37, (2015): 123–32. https://doi.org/10.1016/j.concog.2015.09.001.

Bendich, A. "Physiological Role of Antioxidants in the Immune System." *Journal of Dairy Science* 76, no. 9 (1993): 2789–94. https://doi.org/10.3168/jds.s0022-0302(93)77617-1.

Benzie, Iris F. F., and Sissi Wachtel-Galor, eds. *Herbal Medicine: Biomolecular and Clinical Aspects.* 2nd ed. Florida: CRC Press, 2011.

Bertoglio, Kiah, S. Jill James, Lesley Deprey, Norman Brule, and Robert L. Hendren. "Pilot Study of the Effect of Methyl B12 Treatment on Behavioral and Biomarker Measures in Children with Autism." *The Journal of Alternative and Complementary Medicine* 16, no. 5 (2010a): 555–60. https://doi.org/10.1089/acm.2009.0177.

Besedovsky, Luciana, Tanja Lange, and Jan Born. "Sleep and Immune Function." *Pflügers Archiv - European Journal of Physiology* 463, no. 1 (2011): 121–37. https://doi.org/10.1007/s00424-011-1044-0.

Bested, Alison C., Alan C. Logan, and Eva M. Selhub. "Intestinal Microbiota, Probiotics and Mental Health: From Metchnikoff to Modern Advances: Part II – Contemporary Contextual Research." *Gut Pathogens* 5, no. 1 (2013): 3. https://doi.org/10.1186/1757-4749-5-3.

Bloch, Michael H., and Ahmad Qawasmi. "Omega-3 Fatty Acid Supplementation for the Treatment of Children With Attention-deficit/Hyperactivity Disorder Symptomatology: Systematic Review and Meta-Analysis." *Journal of the American Academy of Child and Adolescent Psychiatry* 50, no. 10, (2011): 991–1000. https://doi.org/10.1016/j.jaac.2011.06.008.

Bloch, Michael H., and Jilian Mulqueen. "Nutritional Supplements for the Treatment of ADHD." *Child and Adolescent Psychiatric Clinics of North America* 23, no. 4 (2014): 883–97. https://doi.org/10.1016/j.chc.2014.05.002.

Boggiss, Anna L., Nathan S. Consedine, Jennifer M. Brenton-Peters, Paul L. Hofman, and Anna S. Serlachius. "A Systematic Review of Gratitude Interventions: Effects on Physical Health and Health Behaviors." *Journal of Psychosomatic Research* 135, (2020): 110165. https://doi.org/10.1016/j.jpsychores.2020.110165.

Boyer, Jeanelle, and Rui Hai Liu. "Apple Phytochemicals and Their Health Benefits." *Nutrition Journal* 3, (2004): 5. https://doi.org/10.1186/1475-2891-3-5.

Brahmachari, Goutam, ed. *Discovery and Development of Anti-Inflammatory Agents from Natural Products.* 1st ed. Vol. 4 of *Natural Product Drug Discovery.* Amsterdam: Elsevier, 2019.

Brambilla, Daria, Cesare Mancuso, Mariagrazia Rita Scuderi, Paolo Bosco, Giuseppina Cantarella, Laurence Lempereur, Giulia Di Benedetto, Salvatore Pezzino, and Renato Bernardini. "The Role of Antioxidant Supplement in Immune System, Neoplastic, and Neurodegenerative Disorders: A Point of View for an Assessment of the Risk/Benefit Profile." *Nutrition Journal* 7, no. 1 (2008): 29. https://doi.org/10.1186/1475-2891-7-29.

Bull-Larsen, Stephanie, and M. Hasan Mohajeri. "The Potential Influence of the Bacterial Microbiome on the Development and Progression of ADHD." *Nutrients* 11, no. 11 (2019): 2805. https://doi.org/10.3390/nu11112805.

Cannell, John Jacob. "Vitamin D and Autism, What's New?" *Reviews in Endocrine and Metabolic Disorders* 18, no. 2 (2017): 183–93. https://doi.org/10.1007/s11154-017-9409-0.

Castro-Rodriguez, Jose A., and Luis Garcia-Marcos. "What Are the Effects of a Mediterranean Diet on Allergies and Asthma in Children?" *Frontiers in Pediatrics* 5, (2017a): 72. https://doi.org/10.3389/fped.2017.00072.

Cefalu, William T. "Achieving Type 2 Diabetes Remission Through Weight Loss."

Diabetes Discoveries & Practice Blog. National Institute of Diabetes and Digestive and Kidney Diseases, September 30, 2020. https://www.niddk.nih.gov/health-information/professionals/diabetes-discoveries-practice/achieving-type-2-diabetes-remission-through-weight-loss.

Cerhan, James R., Kenneth G. Saag, Linda A. Merlino, Ted R Mikuls, and Lindsey A. Criswell. "Antioxidant Micronutrients and Risk of Rheumatoid Arthritis in a Cohort of Older Women." *American Journal of Epidemiology* 157, no. 4 (2003): 345–54. https://doi.org/10.1093/aje/kwf205.

Chang, Kristen. "Nutrition & Immune Health." Virginia Academy of Nutrition and Dietetics. https://eatrightvirginia.org/nutrition-immune-health/.

Chang, Shao-Min, and Chung-Hey Chen. "Effects of an Intervention with Drinking Chamomile Tea on Sleep Quality and Depression in Sleep Disturbed Postnatal Women: A Randomized Controlled Trial." *Journal of Advanced Nursing* 72, no. 2 (2015): 306–15. https://doi.org/10.1111/jan.12836.

Cherpak, Christine E. "Mindful Eating: A Review of How the Stress-digestion Mindfulness Triad May Modulate and Improve Gastrointestinal and Digestive Function." *Integrative Medicine* 18, no. 4 (2019): 48–53. https://pubmed.ncbi.nlm.nih.gov/32549835/.

Chick, Christina F., Anisha Singh, Lauren A. Anker, Casey Buck, Makoto Kawai, Christine Gould, Isabelle Cotto, Logan Schneider, Omer Linkovski, Rosy Karna, Sophia Pirog, Kai Paerker-Fong, Christian R. Nolan, Deanna N. Shinsky, Priynka N. Hiteshi, Oscar Leyva, Brenda Flores, Ryan Matlow, Travis Bradley, Josh Jordan, Victor Carrion, and Ruth O'Hara. "A School-based Health and Mindfulness Curriculum Improves Children's Objectively Measured Sleep." *Sleep* 44, no. 2 (2021): A251–2. https://doi.org/10.1093/sleep/zsab072.640.

Cooper, Ruth E., Charlotte Tye, Jonna Kuntsi, Evangelos Vassos, and Philip Asherson. "The Effect of Omega-3 Polyunsaturated Fatty Acid Supplementation on Emotional Dysregulation, Oppositional Behaviour and Conduct Problems in ADHD: A Systematic Review and Meta-Analysis." *Journal of Affective Disorders* 190, (2016): 474–82. https://doi.org/10.1016/j.jad.2015.09.053.

Das, Rashmi R., Meenu Singh, and Shafiq Nusrat. "Probiotics for Prevention or Treatment of Asthma." *Chest* 138, no. 4 (2010): 307A. https://doi.org/10.1378/chest.9485.

Deledda, Andrea, Giuseppe Annunziata, Gian Carlo Tenore, Vanessa Palmas, Aldo Manzin, and Fernanda Velluzzi. "Diet-derived Antioxidants and Their Role in Inflammation, Obesity and Gut Microbiota Modulation." *Antioxidants* 10, no. 5 (2021): 708. https://doi.org/10.3390/antiox10050708.

Densford, Daryl. "*In the Foxhole (a Soldier's Poem).*" *The Chaplain Kit.* March 25, 2016. https://thechaplainkit.com/2016/03/25/in-the-foxhole-a-soldiers-poem/.

Eaton, Melissa, Joseph Firth, and Jerome Sarris. "Nutrition and Mental Health—How the Food We Eat Can Affect Our Mood." *Frontiers for Young Minds* 8, (2020): 115. https://doi.org/10.3389/frym.2020.00115.

Fedoreyev, Sergey A., Natalia V. Krylova, Natalia P. Mishchenko, Elen A. Vasileva, Evgeny A. Pislyagin, Olga V. Iunikhina, Vyacheslav F. Lavrov, Oksana A. Svitich, Linna K. Ebralidze, and Galina N. Leonova. "Antiviral and Antioxidant Properties of Echinochrome A." *Marine Drugs* 16, no. 12 (2018): 509. https://doi.org/10.3390/md16120509.

Fernandes, Maria, David M. Mutch, and Francesco Leri. "The Relationship Between Fatty Acids and Different Depression-related Brain Regions, and Their Potential Role as Biomarkers of Response to Antidepressants." *Nutrients* 9, no. 3 (2017): 298. https://doi.org/10.3390/nu9030298.

Fristad, Mary A., Anthony T. Vesco, Andrea S. Young, K. Zachary Healy, Elias S. Nader, William Gardner, Adina M. Seidenfeld, Hannah L. Wolfson, and L. Eugene Arnold. "Pilot Randomized Controlled Trial of Omega-3 and Individual Family Psychoeducational Psychotherapy for Children and Adolescents with Depression." *Journal of Clinical Child & Adolescent Psychology* 48, sup. 1 (2016): S105–18. https://doi.org/10.1080/15374416.2016.1233500.

Furushima, Daisuke, Kazuki Ide, and Hiroshi Yamada. "Effect of Tea Catechins on Influenza Infection and the Common Cold with a Focus on Epidemiological/Clinical Studies." *Molecules* 23, no. 7 (2018): 1795. https://doi.org/10.3390/molecules23071795.

Gautam, Medhavi, Mukta Agrawal, Manaswi Gautam, Praveen Sharma, Anita Sharma Gautam, and Shiv Gautam. "Role of Antioxidants in Generalized Anxiety Disorder and Depression." *Indian Journal of Psychiatry* 54, no. 3 (2012): 244. https://doi.org/10.4103/0019-5545.102424.

Gesch, C. Bernard, Sean M. Hammond, Sarah E. Hampson, Anita Eves, and Martin J. Crowder. "Influence of Supplementary Vitamins, Minerals and Essential Fatty Acids on the Antisocial Behaviour of Young Adult Prisoners." *British Journal of Psychiatry* 181, no. 1 (2002): 22–8. https://doi.org/10.1192/bjp.181.1.22.

Gilliland, Frank D., Kiros T. Berhane, Yu-Fen Li, Deborah H. Kim, and Helene G. Margolis. "Dietary Magnesium, Potassium, Sodium, and Children's Lung Function." *American Journal of Epidemiology* 155, no. 2 (2002): 125–31. https://doi.org/10.1093/aje/155.2.125.

Gómez-Pinilla, Fernando. "Brain Foods: The Effects of Nutrients on Brain Function." *Nature Reviews Neuroscience* 9, no. 7 (2008): 568–78. https://doi.org/10.1038/nrn2421.

Griffin, Morgan R. "Natural Cold and Flu Remedies: Americans Are Turning to Cold and Flu Supplements in Greater Numbers." *WebMD*. Reviewed December 29, 2010. https://www.webmd.com/a-to-z-guides/features/colds-flu-immune-system#1.

Guilleminault, Laurent, Evan J. Williams, Hayley A. Scott, Bronwyn S. Berthon, Megan Jensen, and Lisa G. Wood. "Diet and Asthma: Is It Time to Adapt Our Message?" *Nutrients* 9, no. 11 (2017): 1227. https://doi.org/10.3390/nu9111227.

Guillin, Olivia M., Caroline Vindry, Théophile Ohlmann, and Laurent Chavatte. "Selenium, Selenoproteins and Viral Infection." *Nutrients* 11, no. 9 (2019): 2101. https://doi.org/10.3390/nu11092101.

Guo, Ying, Jianping Xie, Xia Li, Yun Yuan, Lanchun Zhang, Weiyan Hu, Haiyun Luo, Haofei Yu, and Rongping Zhang. "Antidepressant Effects of Rosemary Extracts Associate with Anti-inflammatory Effect and Rebalance of Gut Microbiota." *Frontiers in Pharmacology* 9, (2018): 1126. https://doi.org/10.3389/fphar.2018.01126.

Hansen, Anita L., Gina Olson, Lisbeth Dahl, David Thornton, Bjørn Grung, Ingvild E. Graff, Livar Frøyland, and Julian F. Thayer. "Reduced Anxiety in Forensic Inpatients After a Long-term Intervention with Atlantic Salmon." *Nutrients* 6, no. 12 (2014): 5405–18. https://doi.org/10.3390/nu6125405.

Harms, Lauren R., Thomas H. J. Burne, Darryl W. Eyles, and John J. McGrath. "Vitamin D and the Brain." *Best Practice & Research Clinical Endocrinology & Metabolism* 25, no. 4 (2011): 657–69. https://doi.org/10.1016/j.beem.2011.05.009.

Harvard School of Public Health. "Mindful Eating." The Nutrition Source. Posted September 18, 2020. https://www.hsph.harvard.edu/nutritionsource/mindful-eating/.

Haugen, Marilyn, and Doug Cook. *175 Superfood Blender Recipes: Using Your NutriBullet.* Ontario: Robert Rose, 2016.

Hemilä, Harri. "Vitamin C and Community-acquired Pneumonia." *American Journal of Respiratory and Critical Care Medicine* 184, no. 5 (2011): 621–2. https://doi.org/10.1164/ajrccm.184.5.621a.

——. "Zinc Lozenges May Shorten the Duration of Colds: A Systematic Review." *The Open Respiratory Medicine Journal* 5, no. 1 (2011): 51–8. https://doi.org/10.2174/1874306401105010051.

——. "Vitamin C and Infections." *Nutrients* 9, no. 4 (2017): 339. https://doi.org/10.3390/nu9040339.

Henriksen, Danah, Carmen Richardson, and Kyle Shack. "Mindfulness and Creativity: Implications for Thinking and Learning." *Thinking Skills and Creativity* 37, (2020): 100689. https://doi.org/10.1016/j.tsc.2020.100689.

Hewedi, D., G. Mostafa, and E. M. A. N. El Hadidi. "Oxidative Stress in Egyptian Children with Autism: Relation to Autoimmunity." *European Psychiatry* 30, (2015): 807. https://doi.org/10.1016/s0924-9338(15)30628-3.

Hidese, Shinsuke, Shintaro Ogawa, Miho Ota, Ikki Ishida, Zenta Yasukawa, Makoto Ozeki, and Hiroshi Kunugi. "Effects of L-Theanine Administration on Stress-Related Symptoms and Cognitive Functions in Healthy Adults: A Randomized Controlled Trial." *Nutrients* 11, no. 10 (2019): 2362. https://doi.org/10.3390/nu11102362.

Howatson, Glyn, Phillip G. Bell, Jamie Tallent, Benita Middleton, Malachy P. McHugh, and Jason Ellis. "Effect of Tart Cherry Juice (Prunus Cerasus) on Melatonin Levels and Enhanced Sleep Quality." *European Journal of Nutrition* 51, no. 8 (2011): 909–16. https://doi.org/10.1007/s00394-011-0263-7.

Huang, Qingyi, Huan Liu, Katsuhiko Suzuki, Sihui Ma, and Chunhong Liu. "Linking What We Eat to Our Mood: A Review of Diet, Dietary Antioxidants, and Depression." *Antioxidants* 8, no. 9 (2019): 376. https://doi.org/10.3390/antiox8090376.

Huang, Ruixue, Ke Wang, and Jianan Hu. "Effect of Probiotics on Depression: A Systematic Review and Meta-Analysis of Randomized Controlled Trials." *Nutrients* 8, no. 8 (2016): 483. https://doi.org/10.3390/nu8080483.

Huang, Zhiyi, Yu Liu, Guangying Qi, David Brand, and Song Guo Zheng. "Role of Vitamin A in the Immune System." *Journal of Clinical Medicine* 7, no. 9 (2018): 258. https://doi.org/10.3390/jcm7090258.

Iddir, Mohammed, Alex Brito, Giulia Dingeo, Sofia Sosa Fernandez Del Campo, Hanen Samouda, Michael R. La Frano, and Torsten Bohn. "Strengthening the Immune System and Reducing Inflammation and Oxidative Stress through Diet and Nutrition: Considerations During the COVID-19 Crisis." *Nutrients* 12, no. 6 (2020): 1562. https://doi.org/10.3390/nu12061562.

Jacka, Felice N. "Nutritional Psychiatry: Where to Next?" *EBioMedicine* 17, (2017): 24–9. https://doi.org/10.1016/j.ebiom.2017.02.020.

——, Adrienne O'Neil, Rachelle Opie, Catherine Itsiopoulos, Sue Cotton, Mohammedreza Mohebbi, David Castle, Sarah Dash, Cathrine Mihalopoulos, Mary Lou Chatterton, Laima Brazionis, Olivia M. Dean, Allison M. Hodge, and Michael Berk. "A Randomised Controlled Trial of Dietary Improvement for Adults with Major Depression (The 'SMILES' Trial)." *BMC Medicine* 15, no. 1 (2017): 23. https://doi.org/10.1186/s12916-017-0791-y.

James, S. Jill, Stepan Melnyk, George Fuchs, Tyra Reid, Stefanie Jernigan, Oleksandra Pavliv, Amanda Hubanks, and David W. Gaylor. "Efficacy of Methylcobalamin and Folinic Acid Treatment on Glutathione Redox Status in Children with Autism." *The American Journal of Clinical Nutrition* 89, no. 1 (2008): 425–30. https://doi.org/10.3945/ajcn.2008.26615.

Johnson, Elizabeth J., Karen Mcdonald, Susan M. Caldarella, Hae-Yun Chung, Aron M. Troen, and D. Max Snodderly. "Cognitive Findings of an Exploratory Trial of Docosahexaenoic Acid and Lutein Supplementation in Older Women." *Nutritional Neuroscience* 11, no. 2 (2008): 75–83. https://doi.org/10.1179/147683008x301450.

Johnson, Stewart M., and Eric Hollander. "Evidence That Eicosapentaenoic Acid is Effective in Treating Autism." *The Journal of Clinical Psychiatry* 64, no. 7 (2003): 848–9. https://doi.org/10.4088/jcp.v64n0718c.

Jolliffe, David A., Lauren Greenberg, Richard L. Hooper, Christopher J. Griffiths, Carlos A. Camargo, Jr., Conor P. Kerley, Megan E. Jensen, David Mauger, Iwona Stelmach, Mitsuyoshi Urashima, and Adrian R. Martineau. "Vitamin D Supplementation to Prevent Asthma Exacerbations: A Systematic Review and Meta-Analysis of Individual Participant Data." *The Lancet Respiratory Medicine* 5, no. 11 (2017): 881–90. https://doi.org/10.1016/s2213-2600(17)30306-5.

Juszkiewicz, A., A. Glapa, P. Basta, E. Petriczko, K. Żołnowski, B. Machaliński, J. Trzeciak, K. Łuczkowska, and A. Skarpańska-Stejnborn. "The Effect of L-Theanine Supplementation on the Immune System of Athletes Exposed to Strenuous Physical Exercise." *Journal of the International Society of Sports Nutrition* 16, no. 1 (2019): 7. https://doi.org/10.1186/s12970-019-0274-y.

Kalt, Wilhelmina, Aedin Cassidy, Luke R. Howard, Robert Krikorian, April J. Stull, Francois Tremblay, and Raul Zamora-Ros. "Recent Research on the Health Benefits of Blueberries and Their Anthocyanins." *Advances in Nutrition* 11, no. 2 (2020): 224–36. https://doi.org/10.1093/advances/nmz065.

Kanauchi, Osamu, Akira Andoh, Sazaly AbuBakar, and Naoki Yamamoto. "Probiotics and Paraprobiotics in Viral Infection: Clinical Application and Effects on the Innate and Acquired Immune Systems." *Current Pharmaceutical Design* 24, no. 6 (2018): 710–7. https://doi.org/10.2174/1381612824666180116163411.

Kang, En-Jin, Soo Young Kim, In-Hong Hwang, and Yun-Jeong Ji. "The Effect of Probiotics on Prevention of Common Cold: A Meta-Analysis of Randomized Controlled Trial Studies." *Korean Journal of Family Medicine* 34, no. 1 (2013): 2. https://doi.org/10.4082/kjfm.2013.34.1.2.

Keng, Shian-Ling, Moria J. Smoski, and Clive J. Robins. "Effects of Mindfulness on Psychological Health: A Review of Empirical Studies." *Clinical Psychology Review* 31, no. 6 (2011): 1041–56. https://doi.org/10.1016/j.cpr.2011.04.006.

Khalid, Sundus, Katie L. Barfoot, Gabrielle May, Daniel J. Lamport, Shirley A. Reynolds, and Claire M. Williams. "Effects of Acute Blueberry Flavonoids on Mood in Children and Young Adults." *Nutrients* 9, no. 2 (2017): 158. https://doi.org/10.3390/nu9020158.

Kiecolt-Glaser, Janice K., Heather M. Derry, and Christopher P. Fagundes. "Inflammation: Depression Fans the Flames and Feasts on the Heat." *American Journal of Psychiatry* 172, no. 11 (2015): 1075–91. https://doi.org/10.1176/appi.ajp.2015.15020152.

King, Sarah, Julie Glanville, Mary Ellen Sanders, Anita Fitzgerald, and Danielle Varley. "Effectiveness of Probiotics on the Duration of Illness in Healthy Children and Adults Who Develop Common Acute Respiratory Infectious Conditions: A Systematic Review and Meta-Analysis." *British Journal of Nutrition* 112, no. 1 (2014): 41–54. https://doi.org/10.1017/s0007114514000075.

Klemm, Sarah. "Support Your Health with Nutrition." EatRight.Org. Academy of Nutrition and Dietetics. Published December 9, 2019. Reviewed April 2020. https://www.eatright.org/health/wellness/preventing-illness/support-your-health-with-nutrition.

Kodama, Yuzo, Yuki Kishimoto, Yoko Muramatsu, Junko Tatebe, Yu Yamamoto, Nao Hirota, Yukinari Itoigawa, Ryo Atsuta, Kengo Koike, Tadashi Sato, Koich Aizawa, Kazuhisa Takahashi, Toshisuke Morita, Sakae Homma, Kuniaki Seyama, and Akihito Ishigami. "Antioxidant Nutrients in Plasma of Japanese Patients with Chronic Obstructive Pulmonary Disease, Asthma-COPD Overlap Syndrome and Bronchial Asthma." The Clinical Respiratory Journal 11, no. 6 (2016): 915–24. https://doi.org/10.1111/crj.12436.

Kotepui, Manas. "Diet and Risk of Breast Cancer." Współczesna Onkologia 20, no.1 (2016): 13–9. https://doi.org/10.5114/wo.2014.40560.

Kumperscak, Hojka Gregoric, Alja Gricar, Ina ÜLen, and Dusanka Micetic-Turk. "A Pilot Randomized Control Trial with the Probiotic Strain Lactobacillus Rhamnosus GG (LGG) in ADHD: Children and Adolescents Report Better Health-related Quality of Life." Frontiers in Psychiatry 11, (2020): 181. https://doi.org/10.3389/fpsyt.2020.00181.

Lang, Undine E., Christoph Beglinger, Nina Schweinfurth, Marc Walter, and Stefan Borgwardt. "Nutritional Aspects of Depression." Cellular Physiology and Biochemistry 37, no. 3 (2015): 1029–43. https://doi.org/10.1159/000430229.

Larkin, Emma K., Yu-Tang Gao, Tebeb Gebretsadik, Terryl J. Hartman, Pingsheng Wu, Wanqing Wen, Gong Yang, Chunxue Bai, Meiling Jin, L. Jackson Roberts, II, Myron Gross, Xiao O. Shu, and Tina V. Hartert. "New Risk Factors for Adult-Onset Incident Asthma. A Nested Case-Control Study of Host Antioxidant Defense." American Journal of Respiratory and Critical Care Medicine 191, no. 1 (2015): 45–53. https://doi.org/10.1164/rccm.201405-0948oc.

Laursen, Rikke Pilmann, and Iva Hojsak. "Probiotics for Respiratory Tract Infections in Children Attending Day Care Centers-A Systematic Review." European Journal of Pediatrics 177, no. 7 (2018): 979–94. https://doi.org/10.1007/s00431-018-3167-1.

Lee, Clara S. C., Man-Ting Ma, Hin-Yui Ho, Ka-Kei Tsang, Yi-Yi Zheng, and Zou-Yi Wu. "The Effectiveness of Mindfulness-based Intervention in Attention on Individuals with ADHD: A Systematic Review." Hong Kong Journal of Occupational Therapy 30, no. 1 (2017): 33–41. https://doi.org/10.1016/j.hkjot.2017.05.001.

Lehtoranta, L., A. Pitkäranta, and R. Korpela. "Probiotics in Respiratory Virus Infections." European Journal of Clinical Microbiology & Infectious Diseases 33, no. 8 (2014): 1289–302. https://doi.org/10.1007/s10096-014-2086-y.

Li, Yanyan, Tao Zhang, Hasan Korkaya, Suling Liu, Hsiu-Fang Lee, Bryan Newman, Yanke Yu, Shawn G. Clouthier, Steven J. Schwartz, Max S. Wicha, and Duxin Sun. "Sulforaphane, a Dietary Component of Broccoli/Broccoli Sprouts, Inhibits Breast Cancer Stem Cells." Clinical Cancer Research 16, no. 9 (2010): 2580–90. https://doi.org/10.1158/1078-0432.ccr-09-2937.

Li, Ye, Mei-Rong Lv, Yan-Lin Wei, Ling Sun, Ji-Xiang Zhang, Huai-Guo Zhang, and Bin Li. "Dietary Patterns and Depression Risk: A Meta-Analysis." *Psychiatry Research* 253, (2017): 373–82. https://doi.org/10.1016/j.psychres.2017.04.020.

Lien, Lars, Nanna Lien, Sonja Heyerdahl, Magne Thoresen, and Espen Bjertness. "Consumption of Soft Drinks and Hyperactivity, Mental Distress, and Conduct Problems Among Adolescents in Oslo, Norway." *American Journal of Public Health* 96, no. 10 (2006): 1815–20. https://doi.org/10.2105/ajph.2004.059477.

Lima, Leonardo C. R., Renan V. Barreto, Natália M. Bassan, Camila C. Greco, and Benedito S. Denadai. "Consumption of an Anthocyanin-rich Antioxidant Juice Accelerates Recovery of Running Economy and Indirect Markers of Exercise-induced Muscle Damage Following Downhill Running." *Nutrients* 11, no. 10 (2019): 2274. https://doi.org/10.3390/nu11102274.

Liu, Yuying, Jane J. Alookaran, and J. Marc Rhoads. "Probiotics in Autoimmune and Inflammatory Disorders." *Nutrients* 10, no. 10 (2018): 1537. https://doi.org/10.3390/nu10101537.

Louise, Stephanie, Molly Fitzpatrick, Clara Strauss, Susan L. Rossell, and Neil Thomas. "Mindfulness- and Acceptance-based Interventions for Psychosis: Our Current Understanding and a Meta-Analysis." *Schizophrenia Research* 192, (2018): 57–63. https://doi.org/10.1016/j.schres.2017.05.023.

Magalhães, Pedro V. S., Olivia Dean, Ana C. Andreazza, Michael Berk, and Flávio Kapczinski. "Antioxidant Treatments for Schizophrenia." *Cochrane Database of Systematic Reviews* 2, (2016): CD008919. https://doi.org/10.1002/14651858.cd008919.pub2.

Makki, Kassem, Edward C. Deehan, Jens Walter, and Fredrik Bäckhed. "The Impact of Dietary Fiber on Gut Microbiota in Host Health and Disease." *Cell Host & Microbe* 23, no. 6 (2018): 705–15. https://doi.org/10.1016/j.chom.2018.05.012.

Manivasagam, Thamilarasan, Selvaraj Arunadevi, Mustafa Mohamed Essa, Chidambaram SaravanaBabu, Anupom Borah, Arokiasamy Justin Thenmozhi, and M. Walid Qoronfleh. "Role of Oxidative Stress and Antioxidants in Autism." *Advances in Neurobiology* 24, (2020): 193–206. https://doi.org/10.1007/978-3-030-30402-7_7.

Mao, Jun J., Sharon X. Xie, John R. Keefe, Irene Soeller, Qing S. Li, and Jay D. Amsterdam. "Long-term Chamomile (Matricaria Chamomilla L.) Treatment for Generalized Anxiety Disorder: A Randomized Clinical Trial." *Phytomedicine* 23, no. 14 (2016): 1735–42. https://doi.org/10.1016/j.phymed.2016.10.012.

Maroon, Joseph Charles, and Jeffrey W. Bost. "Omega-3 Fatty Acids (Fish Oil) as an Anti-inflammatory: An Alternative to Nonsteroidal Anti-inflammatory Drugs for Discogenic Pain." *Surgical Neurology* 65, no. 4 (2006): 326–31. https://doi.org/10.1016/j.surneu.2005.10.023.

Martin, Francois-Pierre J., Serge Rezzi, Emma Peré-Trepat, Beate Kamlage, Sebastiano Collino, Edgar Leibold, Jürgen Kastler, Dietrich Rein, Laurent B. Fay, and Sunil Kochhar. "Metabolic Effects of Dark Chocolate Consumption on Energy, Gut Microbiota, and Stress-related Metabolism in Free-living Subjects." *Journal of Proteome Research* 8, no. 12 (2009): 5568–79. https://doi.org/10.1021/pr900607v.

Mathee, Kalai, Trevor Cickovski, Alok Deoraj, Melanie Stollstorff, and Giri Narasimhan. "The Gut Microbiome and Neuropsychiatric Disorders: Implications for Attention Deficit Hyperactivity Disorder (ADHD)." *Journal of Medical Microbiology* 69, no. 1 (2020): 14–24. https://doi.org/10.1099/jmm.0.001112.

McCann, Donna, Angelina Barrett, Alison Cooper, Debbie Crumpler, Lindy Dalen, Kate Grimshaw, Elizabeth Kitchin, Kris Lok, Lucy Porteous, Emily Prince, Edmund Sonuga-Barke, John O. Warner, and Jim Stevenson. "Food Additives and Hyperactive Behaviour in 3-Year-Old and 8/9-Year-Old Children in the Community: A Randomised, Double-blinded, Placebo-controlled Trial." *Lancet* 370, no. 9598 (2007): 1560–7. https://doi.org/10.1016/s0140-6736(07)61306-3.

Meguid, Nagwa A., Hazem M. Atta, Amr S. Gouda, and Rehab O. Khalil. "Role of Polyunsaturated Fatty Acids in the Management of Egyptian Children with Autism." *Clinical Biochemistry* 41, no. 13 (2008): 1044–8. https://doi.org/10.1016/j.clinbiochem.2008.05.013.

Mentella, Maria Chiara, Franco Scaldaferri, Caterina Ricci, Antonio Gasbarrini, and Giacinto Abele Donato Miggiano. "Cancer and Mediterranean Diet: A Review." *Nutrients* 11, no. 9 (2019): 2059. https://doi.org/10.3390/nu11092059.

Merriam-Webster, s.v. "bronchiectasis (*n.*)." Accessed July 26, 2021. https://www.merriam-webster.com/dictionary/bronchiectasis.

——, "foxhole (*n.*)." Accessed July 26, 2021. https://www.merriam-webster.com/dictionary/foxhole.

Messaoudi, Michaël, Nicolas Violle, Jean-François Bisson, Didier Desor, Hervé Javelot, and Catherine Rougeot. "Beneficial Psychological Effects of a Probiotic Formulation (Lactobacillus Helveticusr0052 Andbifidobacterium Longumr0175) in Healthy Human Volunteers." *Gut Microbes* 2, no. 4 (2011): 256–61. https://doi.org/10.4161/gmic.2.4.16108.

Messaoudi, Michaël, Robert Lalonde, Nicolas Violle, Hervé Javelot, Didier Desor, Amine Nejdi, Jean-François Bisson, Catherine Rougeot, Matthieu Pichelin, Murielle Cazaubiel, Jean-Marc Cazaubiel. "Assessment of Psychotropic-like Properties of a Probiotic Formulation (Lactobacillus Helveticusr0052 Andbifidobacterium Longumr0175) in Rats and Human Subjects." *British Journal of Nutrition* 105, no. 5 (2010): 755–64. https://doi.org/10.1017/s0007114510004319.

Miki, Takako, Masafumi Eguchi, Kayo Kurotani, Takeshi Kochi, Keisuke Kuwahara, Rie Ito, Yasumi Kimura, Hiroko Tsuruoka, Shamima Akter, Ikuko Kashino, Isamu Kabe, Norito Kawakami, and Tetsuya Mizoue. "Dietary Fiber Intake and Depressive Symptoms in Japanese Employees: The Furukawa Nutrition and Health Study." *Nutrition* 32, no. 5 (2016): 584–9. https://doi.org/10.1016/j.nut.2015.11.014.

Mikirova, N. A., A. M. Rogers, P. R. Taylor, R. E. Hunninghake, J. R. Miranda-Massari, and M. J. Gonzalez. "Metabolic Correction for Attention Deficit/Hyperactivity Disorder: A Biochemical-physiological Therapeutic Approach." *Functional Foods in Health and Disease* 3, no. 1 (2013): 1. https://doi.org/10.31989/ffhd.v3i1.67.

Miller, Marshall G., Derek A. Hamilton, James A. Joseph, and Barbara Shukitt-Hale. "Dietary Blueberry Improves Cognition Among Older Adults in a Randomized, Double-blind, Placebo-controlled Trial." *European Journal of Nutrition* 57, no. 3 (2017): 1169–80. https://doi.org/10.1007/s00394-017-1400-8.

Milte, Catherine M., Natalie Parletta, Jonathan D. Buckley, Alison M. Coates, Ross M. Young, and Peter R. C. Howe. "Eicosapentaenoic and Docosahexaenoic Acids, Cognition, and Behavior in Children with Attention-Deficit/Hyperactivity Disorder: A Randomized Controlled Trial." *Nutrition* 28, no. 6 (2012): 670–7. https://doi.org/10.1016/j.nut.2011.12.009.

Miyata, Jun, and Makoto Arita. "Role of Omega-3 Fatty Acids and Their Metabolites in Asthma and Allergic Diseases." *Allergology International* 64, no. 1 (2015): 27–34. https://doi.org/10.1016/j.alit.2014.08.003.

Mohammadi, Ali Akbar, Shima Jazayeri, Kianoush Khosravi-Darani, Zahra Solati, Nakisa Mohammadpour, Zatollah Asemi, Zohre Adab, Mahmoud Djalali, Mehdi Tehrani-Doost, Mostafa Hosseini, and Shahryar Eghtesadi. "The Effects of Probiotics on Mental Health and Hypothalamic–Pituitary–Adrenal Axis: A Randomized, Double-blind, Placebo-controlled Trial in Petrochemical Workers." *Nutritional Neuroscience* 19, no. 9 (2015): 387–95. https://doi.org/10.1179/1476830515y.0000000023.

Moon, Maggie. *The MIND Diet: A Scientific Approach to Enhancing Brain Function and Helping Prevent Alzheimer's and Dementia.* 1st ed. California: Ulysses Press, 2016.

Mora, J. Rodrigo, Makoto Iwata, and Ulrich H. von Andrian. "Vitamin Effects on the Immune System: Vitamins A and D Take Centre Stage." *Nature Reviews Immunology* 8, no. 9 (2008): 685–98. https://doi.org/10.1038/nri2378.

Mousain-Bosc, M., M. Roche, A. Polge, D. Pradal-Prat, J. Rapin, J. P. Bali. "Improvement of Neurobehavioral Disorders in Children Supplemented with Magnesium-Vitamin B6. I. Attention Deficit Hyperactivity Disorders." *Magnesium Research* 19, no. 1 (2006): 46–52. https://pubmed.ncbi.nlm.nih.gov/16846100/.

Muhammad, Dimas Rahadian Aji, and Koen Dewettinck. "Cinnamon and Its Derivatives as Potential Ingredient in Functional Food—A Review." *International Journal of Food Properties* 20, sup. 2 (2017): 2237–63. https://doi.org/10.1080/10942912.2017.1369102.

Mumme, Karen, and Welma Stonehouse. "Effects of Medium-Chain Triglycerides on Weight Loss and Body Composition: A Meta-Analysis of Randomized Controlled Trials." *Journal of the Academy of Nutrition and Dietetics* 115, no. 2 (2015): 249–63. https://doi.org/10.1016/j.jand.2014.10.022.

Munger, Kassandra L., and Alberto Ascherio. "Prevention and Treatment of MS: Studying the Effects Of Vitamin D." *Multiple Sclerosis Journal* 17, no. 12 (2011): 1405–11. https://doi.org/10.1177/1352458511425366.

Nantz, Meri P., Cheryl A. Rowe, Catherine Muller, Rebecca Creasy, James Colee, Christina Khoo, and Susan S. Percival. "Consumption of Cranberry Polyphenols Enhances Human-T Cell Proliferation and Reduces the Number of Symptoms Associated with Colds and Influenza: A Randomized, Placebo-controlled Intervention Study." *Nutrition Journal* 12, no. 1 (2013): 161. https://doi.org/10.1186/1475-2891-12-161.

National Institutes of Health. "Calcium." Office of Dietary Supplements. Accessed July 31, 2021. https://ods.od.nih.gov/factsheets/Calcium-HealthProfessional/.

National Institutes of Health. "Low Vitamin D Levels Associated with Colds and Flu." NIH Research Matters. Posted April 4, 2016. https://www.nih.gov/news-events/nih-research-matters/low-vitamin-d-levels-associated-colds-flu.

——. "Iron." Office of Dietary Supplements. Accessed July 31, 2021. https://ods.od.nih.gov/factsheets/Iron-Consumer/.

——. "Magnesium." Office of Dietary Supplements. Accessed July 31, 2021. https://ods.od.nih.gov/factsheets/Magnesium-Consumer/.

——. "Potassium." Office of Dietary Supplements. Accessed July 27, 2021. https://ods.od.nih.gov/factsheets/Potassium-HealthProfessional/.

——. "Probiotics: What You Need to Know." National Center for Complementary and Integrative Health. Updated August 2019. https://www.nccih.nih.gov/health/probiotics-what-you-need-to-know.

——. "Vitamin K." Office of Dietary Supplements. Accessed July 31, 2021. https://ods.od.nih.gov/factsheets/vitamink-consumer/.

Navaneenthan, Sankar D., Hans Yehnert, Fady Moustarah, Martin J. Schreiber, Philip R. Schauer, and Srinivasan Beddhu. "Weight Loss Interventions in Chronic Kidney Disease: A Systematic Review and Meta-analysis." *Clinical Journal of the American Society of Nephrology* 4, no. 10 (2009): 1565–1574. https://doi.org/10.2215/cjn.02250409.

Nazir, Yusuf, Syed Ammar Hussain, Aidil Abdul Hamid, and Yuanda Song. "Probiotics and Their Potential Preventive and Therapeutic Role for Cancer, High Serum Cholesterol, and Allergic and HIV Diseases." *BioMed Research International* 2018, ID 3428437 (2018): 1–17. https://doi.org/10.1155/2018/3428437.

Nelson, Joseph B. "Mindful Eating: The Art of Presence While You Eat." *Diabetes Spectrum* 30, no. 3 (2017): 171–4. https://doi.org/10.2337/ds17-0015.

Nematolahi, Pouya, Mitra Mehrabani, Somayyeh Karami-Mohajeri, and Fatemeh Dabaghzadeh. "Effects of Rosmarinus Officinalis L. on Memory Performance, Anxiety, Depression, and Sleep Quality in University Students: A Randomized Clinical Trial." *Complementary Therapies in Clinical Practice* 30, (2018): 24–8. https://doi.org/10.1016/j.ctcp.2017.11.004.

Ng, Qin Xiang, Wayren Loke, Nandini Venkatanarayanan, Donovan Yutong Lim, Alex Yu Sen Soh, and Wee Song Yeo. "A Systematic Review of the Role of Prebiotics and Probiotics in Autism Spectrum Disorders." *Medicina* 55, no. 5 (2019): 129. https://doi.org/10.3390/medicina55050129.

Nieman, David C., Dru A. Henson, Sarah J. Gross, David P. Jenkins, J. Mark Davis, E. Angela Murphy, Martin D. Carmichael, Charles L. Dumke, Alan C. Utter, Steven R. McAnulty, Lisa S. McAnulty, and Eugene P. Mayer. "Quercetin Reduces Illness but Not Immune Perturbations after Intensive Exercise." *Medicine & Science in Sports & Exercise* 39, no. 9 (2007): 1561–9. https://doi.org/10.1249/mss.0b013e318076b566.

Nigg, Joel T., and Kathleen Holton. "Restriction and Elimination Diets in ADHD Treatment." *Child and Adolescent Psychiatric Clinics of North America* 23, no. 4 (2014): 937–53. https://doi.org/10.1016/j.chc.2014.05.010.

O'Neil, Adrienne, Shae E. Quirk, Siobhan Housden, Sharon L. Brennan, Lana J. Williams, Julie A. Pasco, Michael Berk, and Felice N. Jacka. "Relationship Between Diet and Mental Health in Children and Adolescents: A Systematic Review." *American Journal of Public Health* 104, no. 10 (2014): e31–42. https://doi.org/10.2105/ajph.2014.302110.

Opie, Rachelle S., Adrienne O'Neil, Felice N. Jacka, Josephine Pizzinga, and Catherine Itsiopoulos. "A Modified Mediterranean Dietary Intervention for Adults with Major Depression: Dietary Protocol and Feasibility Data from the SMILES Trial." *Nutritional Neuroscience* 21, no. 7 (2017): 487–501. https://doi.org/10.1080/1028415x.2017.1312841.

Pärtty, Anna, Marko Kalliomäki, Pirjo Wacklin, Seppo Salminen, and Erika Isolauri. "A Possible Link Between Early Probiotic Intervention and the Risk of Neuropsychiatric Disorders Later in Childhood: A Randomized Trial." *Pediatric Research* 77, no. 6 (2015): 823–8. https://doi.org/10.1038/pr.2015.51.

Payne, Martha E., Susan E. Steck, Rebecca R. George, and David C. Steffens. "Fruit, Vegetable, and Antioxidant Intakes Are Lower in Older Adults with Depression." *Journal of the Academy of Nutrition and Dietetics* 112, no. 12 (2012): 2022–7. https://doi.org/10.1016/j.jand.2012.08.026.

Pelsser, Lidy M., Klaas Frankena, Jan Toorman, Huub F. Savelkoul, Anthony E. Dubois, Rob Rodrigues Pereira, Ton A. Haagen, Nanda N. Rommelse, and Jan K. Buitelaar. "Effects of a Restricted Elimination Diet on the Behaviour of Children with Attention-Deficit Hyperactivity Disorder (INCA Study): A Randomised Controlled Trial." *Lancet* 377, no. 9764 (2011): 494–503. https://doi.org/10.1016/s0140-6736(10)62227-1.

Perrier, C., and B. Corthésy. "Gut Permeability and Food Allergies." *Clinical & Experimental Allergy* 41, no. 1 (2010): 20–8. https://doi.org/10.1111/j.1365-2222.2010.03639.x.

Peterson, Christine Tara, Dmitry A. Rodionov, Andrei L. Osterman, and Scott N. Peterson. "B Vitamins and Their Role in Immune Regulation and Cancer." *Nutrients* 12, no. 11 (2020): 3380. https://doi.org/10.3390/nu12113380.

Peterson, Michael J., and Ruth M. Benca. "Sleep in Mood Disorders." *Psychiatric Clinics of North America* 29, no. 4 (2006): 1009–32. https://doi.org/10.1016/j.psc.2006.09.003.

Pham, Ngoc Minh, Akiko Nanri, Kayo Kurotani, Keisuke Kuwahara, Ayami Kume, Masao Sato, Hitomi Hayabuchi, and Tetsuya Mizoue. "Green Tea and Coffee Consumption is Inversely Associated with Depressive Symptoms in a Japanese Working Population." *Public Health Nutrition* 17, no. 3 (2013): 625–33. https://doi.org/10.1017/s1368980013000360.

Pierre, Joseph F., Reinhard Hinterleitner, Romain Bouziat, Nathan A. Hubert, Vanessa Leone, Jun Miyoshi, Bana Jabri, and Eugene B. Chang. "Dietary Antioxidant Micronutrients Alter Mucosal Inflammatory Risk in a Murine Modelof Genetic and Microbial Susceptibility." *The Journal of Nutritional Biochemistry* 54, (2018): 95–104. https://doi.org/10.1016/j.jnutbio.2017.12.002.

Plaza-Díaz, Julio, Francisco Javier Ruiz-Ojeda, Laura Maria Vilchez-Padial, and Angel Gil. "Evidence of the Anti-Inflammatory Effects of Probiotics and Synbiotics in Intestinal Chronic Diseases." *Nutrients* 9, no. 6 (2017): 555. https://doi.org/10.3390/nu9060555.

Ptomey, Lauren T., Felicia L. Steger, Matthew M. Schubert, Jaehoon Lee, Erik A. Willis, Debra K. Sullivan, Amanda N. Szabo-Reed, Richard A. Washburn, and Joseph E. Donnelly. "Breakfast Intake and Composition Is Associated with Superior Academic Achievement in Elementary Schoolchildren." *Journal of the American College of Nutrition* 35, no. 4 (2015): 326–33. https://doi.org/10.1080/07315724.2015.1048381.

Puertollano, María A., Elena Puertollano, Gerardo Álvarez de Cienfuegos, and Manuel A. de Pablo. "Dietary Antioxidants: Immunity and Host Defense." *Current Topics in Medicinal Chemistry* 11, no. 14 (2011): 1752–66. https://doi.org/10.2174/156802611796235107.

Quirk, Shae E., Lana J. Williams, Adrienne O'Neil, Julie A. Pasco, Felice N. Jacka, Siobhan Housden, Michael Berk, and Sharon L. Brennan. "The Association Between Diet Quality, Dietary Patterns and Depression in Adults: A Systematic Review." *BMC Psychiatry* 13, no. 1 (2013): 175. https://doi.org/10.1186/1471-244x-13-175.

Rahmani, Ghazal, Fereshteh Farajdokht, Gisou Mohaddes, Shirin Babri, Vida Ebrahimi, and Hadi Ebrahimi. "Garlic (Allium Sativum) Improves Anxiety- and Depressive-related Behaviors and Brain Oxidative Stress in Diabetic Rats." *Archives of Physiology and Biochemistry* 126, no. 2 (2018): 95–100. https://doi.org/10.1080/13813455.2018.1494746.

Redwine, Laura S., Brook L. Henry, Meredith A. Pung, Kathleen Wilson, Kelly Chinh, Brian Knight, Shamini Jain, Thomas Rutledge, Barry Greenberg, Alan Maisel, and Paul J. Mills. "Pilot Randomized Study of a Gratitude Journaling Intervention on Heart Rate Variability and Inflammatory Biomarkers in Patients With Stage B Heart Failure." *Psychosomatic Medicine* 78, no. 6 (2016): 667–76. https://doi.org/10.1097/psy.0000000000000316.

Richette, Pascal, Christine Poitou, Patrick Garnero, Eric Vicaut, Jean-Luc Bouillot, Jean-Marc Lacorte, Arnaud Basdevant, Karine Clément, Thomas Bardin, and Xavier Chevalier. "Benefits of Massive Weight Loss on Symptoms, Systemic Inflammation and Cartilage Turnover in Obese Patients With Knee Osteoarthritis." *BMJ Journals* 70, no. 1 (2011): 139–144. https://doi.org/10.1136/ard.2010.134015.

Ríos-Hernández, Alejandra, José A. Alda, Andreu Farran-Codina, Estrella Ferreira-García, and Maria Izquierdo-Pulido. "The Mediterranean Diet and ADHD in Children and Adolescents." *Pediatrics* 139, no. 2 (2017): e20162027. https://doi.org/10.1542/peds.2016-2027.

Rishikof, Dianne. *Health Takes Guts*. Self-published, 2018, Kindle.

Roman, Pablo, Angeles F. Estévez, Alonso Miras, Nuria Sánchez-Labraca, Fernando Cañadas, Ana B. Vivas, and Diana Cardona. "A Pilot Randomized Controlled Trial to Explore Cognitive and Emotional Effects of Probiotics in Fibromyalgia." *Scientific Reports* 8, no. 1 (2018): 10965. https://doi.org/10.1038/s41598-018-29388-5.

Rondanelli, Mariangela, Alessandro Miccono, Silvia Lamburghini, Ilaria Avanzato, Antonella Riva, Pietro Allegrini, Milena Anna Faliva, Gabriella Peroni, Mara Nichetti, and Simone Perna. "Self-care for Common Colds: The Pivotal Role of Vitamin D, Vitamin C, Zinc, and Echinacea in Three Main Immune Interactive Clusters (Physical Barriers, Innate and Adaptive Immunity) Involved during an Episode of Common Colds—Practical Advice on Dosages and on the Time to Take These Nutrients/Botanicals in order to Prevent or Treat Common Colds." *Evidence-Based Complementary and Alternative Medicine* 2018, (2018): 1–36. https://doi.org/10.1155/2018/5813095.

Rucklidge, Julia J., and Rachel Harrison. "Successful Treatment of Bipolar Disorder II and ADHD with a Micronutrient Formula: A Case Study." *CNS Spectrums* 15, no. 5 (2010): 289–95. https://doi.org/10.1017/s1092852900027516.

Rumble, Meredith E., Kaitlin Hanley White, and Ruth M. Benca. "Sleep Disturbances in Mood Disorders." *Psychiatric Clinics of North America* 38, no. 4 (2015): 743–59. https://doi.org/10.1016/j.psc.2015.07.006.

Saghafian, Faezeh, Hanieh Malmir, Parvane Saneei, Alireza Milajerdi, Bagher Larijani, and Ahmad Esmaillzadeh. "Fruit and Vegetable Consumption and Risk of Depression: Accumulative Evidence from an Updated Systematic Review and Meta-Analysis of Epidemiological Studies." *British Journal of Nutrition* 119, no. 10 (2018): 1087–101. https://doi.org/10.1017/s0007114518000697.

Sakamoto, Filipe Lopes, Rodrigo Metzker Pereira Ribeiro, Allain Amador Bueno, and Heitor Oliveira Santos. "Psychotropic Effects Of L-Theanine and Its Clinical Properties: From the Management of Anxiety and Stress to a Potential Use in Schizophrenia." *Pharmacological Research* 147, (2019): 104395. https://doi.org/10.1016/j. phrs.2019.104395.

Salim, Samina, Gaurav Chugh, and Mohammad Asghar. "Inflammation in Anxiety." *Advances in Protein Chemistry and Structural Biology* Volume 88, (2012): 1–25. https://doi.org/10.1016/b978-0-12-398314-5.00001-5.

Salz, Alyssa. "Substance Abuse and Nutrition." *Today's Dietitian* 16, no. 12 (2014): 44. https://www.todaysdietitian.com/newarchives/120914p44.shtml.

Samuelsen, Anne Berit C., Jürgen Schrezenmeir, and Svein H. Knutsen. "Effects of Orally Administered Yeast-Derived Beta-Glucans: A Review." *Molecular Nutrition & Food Research* 58, no. 1 (2013): 183–93. https://doi.org/10.1002/mnfr.201300338.

Sand, Ilana Katz. "The Role of Diet in Multiple Sclerosis: Mechanistic Connections and Current Evidence." *Current Nutrition Reports* 7, no. 3 (2018): 150–60. https://doi. org/10.1007/s13668-018-0236-z.

Sarris, Jerome, Alan C. Logan, Tasnime N. Akbaraly, G. Paul Amminger, Vicent Balanzá-Martínez, Marlene P. Freeman, Joseph Hibbeln, Yutaka Matsuoka, David Mischoulon, Tetsuya Mizoue, Akiko Nanri, Daisuke Nishi, Drew Ramsey, Julia J. Rucklidge, Almundena Sanchez-Villegas, Andrew Scholey, Kuan-Pin Su, and Felice N. Jacka. "Nutritional Medicine as Mainstream in Psychiatry." *The Lancet Psychiatry* 2, no. 3 (2015): 271–4. https://doi.org/10.1016/s2215-0366(14)00051-0.

Sathyanarayana Rao, T. S., M. R. Asha, B. N. Ramesh, K. S. Jagannatha Rao. "Understanding Nutrition, Depression and Mental Illnesses." *Indian Journal of Psychiatry* 50, no. 2 (2008): 77. https://doi.org/10.4103/0019-5545.42391.

Schauer, Daniel P., Heather Spencer Feigelson, Corinna Koebnick, Bette Caan, Sheila Weinmann, Anthony C. Leonard, J. David Powers, Panduranga R. Yenumula, and David E. Arterburn. "Association Between Weight Loss and the Risk of Cancer After Bariatric Surgery." *The Obesity Society* 25, no. S2 (2017): S52–7. https://doi. org/10.1002/oby.22002

Schneiderman, Neil, Gail Ironson, and Scott D. Siegel. "Stress and Health: Psychological, Behavioral, and Biological Determinants." *Annual Review of Clinical Psychology* 1, no. 1 (2005): 607–28. https://doi.org/10.1146/annurev. clinpsy.1.102803.144141.

Schütz, Katrin, Matthias Sass, Axel de With, Hans-Joachim Graubaum, and Jörg Grünwald. "Immune-modulating Efficacy of a Polyphenol-rich Beverage on Symptoms Associated with the Common Cold: A Double-blind, Randomised, Placebo-controlled, Multi-Centric Clinical Study." *British Journal of Nutrition* 104, no. 8 (2010): 1156–64. https://doi.org/10.1017/s0007114510002047.

Sciutto, Mark J., Denise A. Veres, Tovia L. Marinstein, Brooke F. Bailey, and Sarah K. Cehelyk. "Effects of a School-based Mindfulness Program for Young Children." *Journal of Child and Family Studies* 30, (2021): 1516–27. https://doi.org/10.1007/s10826-021-01955-x.

Sgarbanti, Rossella, Donatella Amatore, Ignacio Celestino, Maria Elena Marcocci, Alessandra Fraternale, Maria Rose Ciriolo, Mauro Magnani, Raffaele Saladino, Enrico Garaci, Anna Teresa Palamara, and Lucia Nencioni. "Intracellular Redox State as Target for Anti-Influenza Therapy: Are Antioxidants Always Effective?" *Current Topics in Medicinal Chemistry* 14, no. 22 (2014): 2529–41. https://doi.org/10.2174/15680266 14666141203125211.

Shaaban, Sanaa Y., Yasmin G. El Gendy, Nayra S. Mehanna, Waled M. El-Senousy, Howaida S. A. El-Feki, Khaled Saad, and Osama M. El-Asheer. "The Role of Probiotics in Children with Autism Spectrum Disorder: A Prospective, Open-Label Study." *Nutritional Neuroscience* 21, no. 9 (2017): 676–81. https://doi.org/10.1080/102841 5x.2017.1347746.

Shankar, A. H., and A. S. Prasad. "Zinc and Immune Function: The Biological Basis of Altered Resistance to Infection." *The American Journal of Clinical Nutrition* 68, no. 2 (1998): 447S–63S. https://doi.org/10.1093/ajcn/68.2.447s.

Sheng, Jia-Ling, Yan Yan, Xiang-Hong Yang, Ti-Fei Yuan, and Dong-Hong Cui. "The Effects of Mindfulness Meditation on Hallucination and Delusion in Severe Schizophrenia Patients with More Than 20 Years' Medical History." *CNS Neuroscience & Therapeutics* 25, no. 1 (2018): 147–50. https://doi.org/10.1111/cns.13067.

Sherry, Amelia R. "Vitamin B12." *Today's Dietitian* 16, no 8 (2014): 20. https://www.todaysdietitian.com/newarchives/080114p20.shtml.

Simopoulos, A. P. "The Importance of the Ratio of Omega-6/Omega-3 Essential Fatty Acids." *Biomedicine & Pharmacotherapy* 56, no. 8 (2002): 365–79. https://doi.org/10.1016/s0753-3322(02)00253-6.

Singh, Meenu, and Rashmi R. Das. "Zinc for the Common Cold." *Cochrane Database of Systematic Reviews*, no. 6 (2013): CD001364. https://doi.org/10.1002/14651858.cd001364.pub4.

Sinn, Natalie, and Janet Bryan. "Effect of Supplementation with Polyunsaturated Fatty Acids and Micronutrients on Learning and Behavior Problems Associated with Child ADHD." *Journal of Developmental & Behavioral Pediatrics* 28, no. 2 (2007): 82–91. https://doi.org/10.1097/01.dbp.0000267558.88457.a5.

Somerville, Vaughan S., Andrea J. Braakhuis, and Will G. Hopkins. "Effect of Flavonoids on Upper Respiratory Tract Infections and Immune Function: A Systematic Review and Meta-Analysis." *Advances in Nutrition* 7, no. 3 (2016): 488–97. https://doi.org/10.3945/an.115.010538.

Spedding, Simon. "Vitamin D and Depression: A Systematic Review and Meta-Analysis Comparing Studies with and without Biological Flaws." *Nutrients* 6, no. 4 (2014): 1501–18. https://doi.org/10.3390/nu6041501.

Stoodley, Isobel, Manohar Garg, Hayley Scott, Lesley Macdonald-Wicks, Bronwyn Berthon, and Lisa Wood. "Higher Omega-3 Index Is Associated with Better Asthma Control and Lower Medication Dose: A Cross-sectional Study." *Nutrients* 12, no. 1 (2019): 74. https://doi.org/10.3390/nu12010074.

Strauss, Clara, Kate Cavanagh, Annie Oliver, and Danelle Pettman. "Mindfulness-Based Interventions for People Diagnosed with a Current Episode of an Anxiety or Depressive Disorder: A Meta-Analysis of Randomised Controlled Trials." *PLoS ONE* 9, no. 4 (2014): e96110. https://doi.org/10.1371/journal.pone.0096110.

Su, Kuan-Pin, Yutaka Matsuoka, and Chi-Un Pae. "Omega-3 Polyunsaturated Fatty Acids in Prevention of Mood and Anxiety Disorders." *Clinical Psychopharmacology and Neuroscience* 13, no. 2 (2015): 129–37. https://doi.org/10.9758/cpn.2015.13.2.129.

Synder, Rachel. "Foxhole Prayers and Why God Is Not Like the Mafia." *ChurchLeaders* (blog), March 20, 2012. https://churchleaders.com/worship/worship-articles/159208-foxhole-prayers-and-why-god-is-not-like-the-mafia.html.

Tabucanon, Thida, Jennifer Wilcox, and W. H. Wilson Tang. "Does Weight Loss Improve Clinical Outcomes in Overweight and Obese Patients with Heart Failure?" *Current Diabetes Reports* 20, no. 75 (2020). https://doi.org/10.1007/s11892-020-01367-z.

Takada, M., K. Nishida, A. Kataoka-Kato, Y Gondo, H. Ishikawa, K. Suda, M. Kawai, R. Hoshi, O. Watanabe, T. Igarashi, Y. Kuwano, K. Miyazaki, and K. Rokutan. "Probiotic Lactobacillus Casei Strain Shirota Relieves Stress-associated Symptoms by Modulating the Gut-Brain Interaction in Human and Animal Models." *Neurogastroenterology & Motility* 28, no. 7 (2016): 1027–36. https://doi.org/10.1111/nmo.12804.

Thushara, Ram Mohan, Surendiran Gangadaran, Zahra Solati, and Mohammed H. Moghadasian. "Cardiovascular Benefits of Probiotics: A Review of Experimental and Clinical Studies." *Food & Function* 7, no. 2 (2016): 632–42. https://doi.org/10.1039/c5fo01190f.

Uebanso, Takashi, Takaaki Shimohata, Kazuaki Mawatari, and Akira Takahashi. "Functional Roles of B Vitamins in the Gut and Gut Microbiome." *Molecular Nutrition & Food Research* 64, no. 18 (2020): 2000426. https://doi.org/10.1002/mnfr.202000426.

Unno, Keiko, Ayane Hara, Aimi Nakagawa, Kazuaki Iguchi, Megumi Ohshio, Akio Morita, and Yoriyuki Nakamura. "Anti-stress Effects of Drinking Green Tea with Lowered Caffeine and Enriched Theanine, Epigallocatechin and Arginine on Psychosocial Stress Induced Adrenal Hypertrophy in Mice." *Phytomedicine*, 23, no. 12 (2016): 1365–74. https://doi.org/10.1016/j.phymed.2016.07.006.

——, Daisuke Furushima, Shingo Hamamoto, Kazuaki Iguchi, Hiroshi Yamada, Akio Morita, Hideki Horie, and Yoriyuki Nakamura. "Stress-reducing Function of Matcha Green Tea in Animal Experiments and Clinical Trials." *Nutrients* 10, no. 10 (2018): 1468. https://doi.org/10.3390/nu10101468.

——, Shigenori Noda, Yohei Kawasaki, Hiroshi Yamada, Akio Morita, Kazuaki Iguchi, and Yoriyuki Nakamura. "Reduced Stress and Improved Sleep Quality Caused by Green Tea Are Associated with a Reduced Caffeine Content." *Nutrients* 9, no. 7 (2017): 777. https://doi.org/10.3390/nu9070777.

Vadell, Anna K. E., Linnea Bärebring, Erik Hulander, Inger Gjertsson, Helen M. Lindqvist, and Anna Winkvist. "Anti-inflammatory Diet in Rheumatoid Arthritis (ADIRA)—A Randomized, Controlled Crossover Trial Indicating Effects on Disease Activity." *The American Journal of Clinical Nutrition* 111, no. 6 (2020): 1203–13. https://doi.org/10.1093/ajcn/nqaa019.

Verkhratsky, Alexei, Maiken Nedergaard, Luca Steardo, and Baoman Li. "Editorial: Sleep and Mood Disorders." *Frontiers in Psychiatry* 10, (2020): 981. https://doi.org/10.3389/fpsyt.2019.00981.

Verlaet, Annelies A., Carlijn M. Maasakkers, Nina Hermans, and Huub F. J. Savelkoul. "Rationale for Dietary Antioxidant Treatment of ADHD." *Nutrients* 10, no. 4 (2018): 405. https://doi.org/10.3390/nu10040405.

Vighi, G., F. Marcucci, L. Sensi, G. Di Cara, and F. Frati. "Allergy and the Gastrointestinal System." *Clinical & Experimental Immunology* 153, suppl. 1 (2008): 3–6. https://doi.org/10.1111/j.1365-2249.2008.03713.x.

Vogel, Jody A., Barry A. Franklin, Kerstyn C. Zalesin, Justin E. Trivax, Kevin R. Krause, David L. Chengelis, and Peter A. McCullough. "Reduction in Predicted Coronary Heart Disease Risk After Substantial Weight Reduction After Bariatric Surgery." *The American Journal of Cardiology* 99, no. 2 (2007): 222–6. https://doi.org/10.1016/j.amjcard.2006.08.017.

Wachtel-Galor, Sissi. *Herbal Medicine: Biomolecular and Clinical Aspects*. 2nd ed. Florida: CRC Press, 2011.

Wang, Yizhong, Xiaolu Li, Ting Ge, Yongmei Xiao, Yang Liao, Yun Cui, Yucai Zhang, Wenzhe Ho, Guangjun Yu, and Ting Zhang. "Probiotics for Prevention and Treatment of Respiratory Tract Infections in Children." *Medicine* 95, no. 31 (2016): e4509. https://doi.org/10.1097/md.0000000000004509.

Webb, Densie. "Herbs and Spices: Holiday Spices." *Today's Dietitian* 18, no. 11 (November 2016), 14. https://www.todaysdietitian.com/newarchives/1116p14.shtml.

Weber, Wendy, and Sanford Newmark. "Complementary and Alternative Medical Therapies for Attention-Deficit/Hyperactivity Disorder and Autism." *Pediatric Clinics of North America* 54, no. 6 (2007): 983–1006. https://doi.org/10.1016/j.pcl.2007.09.006.

WebMD Diet & Weight Management. "Foods High in B Vitamins." Reviewed on December 14, 2020. https://www.webmd.com/diet/foods-high-in-b-vitamins#1.

WebMD. "Beta-Glucans: Uses, Side Effects, and More." Overview. Accessed July 31, 2021. https://www.webmd.com/vitamins/ai/ingredientmono-1041/beta-glucans.

Wright, K. C. "Clinical Nutrition: Beyond Food and Mood." *Today's Dietitian* 21, no. 7 (2019): 10. https://www.todaysdietitian.com/newarchives/0719p10.shtml.

Xie, Zizhen, Fei Chen, William A. Li, Xiaokun Geng, Changhong Li, Xiaomei Meng, Yan Feng, Wei Liu, and Fengchun Yu. "A Review of Sleep Disorders and Melatonin." *Neurological Research* 39, no. 6 (2017): 559–65. https://doi.org/10.1080/01616412.2017.13 15864.

Xue, Jiaming, Yun Zhang, and Ying Huang. "A Meta-Analytic Investigation of the Impact of Mindfulness-based Interventions on ADHD Symptoms." *Medicine* 98, no. 23 (2019): e15957. https://doi.org/10.1097/md.0000000000015957.

Yang, Yang, Long-Gang Zhao, Qi-Jun Wu, Xiao Ma, and Yong-Bing Xiang. "Association Between Dietary Fiber and Lower Risk of All-Cause Mortality: A Meta-Analysis of Cohort Studies." *American Journal of Epidemiology* 181, no. 2 (2015): 83–91. https://doi.org/10.1093/aje/kwu257.

Young, Andrea S., L. Eugene Arnold, Hannah L. Wolfson, and Mary A. Fristad. "Psychoeducational Psychotherapy and Omega-3 Supplementation Improve Co-Occurring Behavioral Problems in Youth with Depression: Results from a Pilot RCT." *Journal of Abnormal Child Psychology* 45, no. 5 (2016): 1025–37. https://doi.org/10.1007/s10802-016-0203-3.

Zeidan, Fadel, Susan K. Johnson, Bruce J. Diamond, Zhanna David, and Paula Goolkasian. "Mindfulness Meditation Improves Cognition: Evidence of Brief Mental Training." *Consciousness and Cognition* 19, no. 2 (2010): 597–605. https://doi.org/10.1016/j.concog.2010.03.014.

Zhao, William, His-En Ho, and Supinda Bunyavanich. "The Gut Microbiome in Food Allergy." *Annals of Allergy, Asthma & Immunology* 122, no. 3 (2019): 276–82. https://doi.org/10.1016/j.anai.2018.12.012.

ADDITIONAL READING

Alramadhan, Elham, Mirna S. Hanna, Mena S. Hanna, Todd A. Goldstein, Samantha M. Avila, and Benjamin S. Weeks. "Dietary and Botanical Anxiolytics." *Medical Science Monitor* 18, no. 4 (2012): RA40–8. https://doi.org/10.12659/msm.882608.

Andrade, Joana M., Célia Faustino, Catarina Garcia, Diogo Ladeiras, Catarina P. Reis, and Patrícia Rijo. "*Rosmarinus Officinalis* L.: An Update Review of Its Phytochemistry and Biological Activity." *Future Science* OA 4, no. 4 (2018a): FSO283. https://doi.org/10.4155/fsoa-2017-0124.

Arreola, Rodrigo, Saray Quintero-Fabián, Rocío Ivette López-Roa, Enrique Octavio Flores-Gutiérrez, Juan Pablo Reyes-Grajeda, Lucrecia Carrera-Quintanar, and Daniel Ortuño-Sahagún. "Immunomodulation and Anti-Inflammatory Effects of Garlic Compounds." *Journal of Immunology Research* 2015, (2015): 1–13. https://doi.org/10.1155/2015/401630.

Braga, Vinícius Lopes, Luana Pompeu Dos Santos Rocha, Daniel Damasceno Bernardo, Carolina de Oliveira Cruz, and Rachel Riera. "What Do Cochrane Systematic Reviews Say About Probiotics as Preventive Interventions?" *Sao Paulo Medical Journal* 135, no. 6 (2017): 578–86. https://doi.org/10.1590/1516-3180.2017.0310241017.

Calder, P. C., and P. Yaqoob. "Glutamine and the Immune System." *Amino Acids* 17, no. 3 (1999): 227–41. https://doi.org/10.1007/bf01366922.

Chang, Jung San, Kuo Chih Wang, Chia Feng Yeh, Den En Shieh, and Lien Chai Chiang. "Fresh Ginger (Zingiber Officinale) Has Anti-viral Activity Against Human Respiratory Syncytial Virus in Human Respiratory Tract Cell Lines." *Journal of Ethnopharmacology* 145, no. 1 (2013): 146–51. https://doi.org/10.1016/j.jep.2012.10.043.

Elder, Jennifer Harrison. "The Gluten-free, Casein-free Diet in Autism: An Overview with Clinical Implications." *Nutrition in Clinical Practice* 23, no. 6 (2008): 583–8. https://doi.org/10.1177/0884533608326061.

Fuglsang, G., G. Madsen, S. Halken, S. Jørgensen, P. A. Ostergaard, and O. Osterballe. "Adverse Reactions to Food Additives in Children with Atopic Symptoms." *Allergy* 49, no. 1 (1994): 31–7. https://doi.org/10.1111/j.1398-9995.1994.tb00770.x.

Gilling, D. H., M. Kitajima, J. R. Torrey, and K. R. Bright. "Antiviral Efficacy and Mechanisms of Action of Oregano Essential Oil and Its Primary Component Carvacrol Against Murine Norovirus." *Journal of Applied Microbiology* 116, no. 5 (2014): 1149–63. https://doi.org/10.1111/jam.12453.

Gray, Paul E. A., Sam Mehr, Constance H. Katelaris, Brynn K. Wainstein, Anita Star, Dianne Campbell, Preeti Joshi, Melanie Wong, Brad Frankum, Karuna Keat, Geraldine Dunne, Barbara Dennison, Alyson Kakakios, and John B. Ziegler. "Salicylate Elimination Diets in Children: Is Food Restriction Supported by the Evidence?" *The Medical Journal of Australia* 198, no. 11 (2013): 600–2. https://doi.org/10.5694/mja12.11255.

Hayashi, K., N. Imanishi, Y. Kashiwayama, A. Kawano, K. Terasawa, Y. Shimada, and H. Ochiai. "Inhibitory Effect of Cinnamaldehyde, Derived from Cinnamomi Cortex, on the Growth of Influenza A/PR/8 Virus in Vitro and in Vivo." *Antiviral Research* 74, no. 1 (2007): 1–8. https://doi.org/10.1016/j.antiviral.2007.01.003.

Hazlewood, Leia C., Lisa G. Wood, Philip M. Hansbro, and Paul S. Foster. "Dietary Lycopene Supplementation Suppresses Th2 Responses and Lung Eosinophilia in a Mouse Model of Allergic Asthma." *The Journal of Nutritional Biochemistry* 22, no. 1(2011): 95–100. https://doi.org/10.1016/j.jnutbio.2009.12.003.

Jesenak, Milos, Ingrid Urbancikova, and Peter Banovcin. "Respiratory Tract Infections and the Role of Biologically Active Polysaccharides in Their Management and Prevention." *Nutrients* 9, no. 7 (2017): 779. https://doi.org/10.3390/nu9070779.

Jia, Kai, Xin Tong, Rong Wang, and Xin Song. "The Clinical Effects of Probiotics for Inflammatory Bowel Disease." *Medicine* 97, no. 51 (2018): e13792. https://doi.org/10.1097/md.0000000000013792.

Josling, P. "Preventing the Common Cold with a Garlic Supplement: A Double-blind, Placebo-controlled Survey." *Advances in Therapy* 18, no. 4 (2001): 189–93. https://doi.org/10.1007/bf02850113.

Kemmerich, Bernd, Reinhild Eberhardt, and Holger Stammer. "Efficacy and Tolerability of a Fluid Extract Combination of Thyme Herb and Ivy Leaves and Matched Placebo in Adults Suffering from Acute Bronchitis with Productive Cough." *Arzneimittelforschung* 56, no. 9 (2011): 652–60. https://doi.org/10.1055/s-0031-1296767.

Kemp, A. "Food additives and hyperactivity." *BMJ* 336, no. 7654 (2008): 1144. https://doi.org/10.1136/bmj.39582.375336.be.

Kennedy, David O., Sonia Pace, Crystal Haskell, Edward J. Okello, Anthea Milne, and Andrew B. Scholey. "Effects of Cholinesterase Inhibiting Sage (Salvia officinalis) on Mood, Anxiety and Performance on a Psychological Stressor Battery." *Neuropsychopharmacology* 31, no. 4 (2005): 845–52. https://doi. org/10.1038/sj.npp.1300907.

Konofal, Eric, Michel Lecendreux, Isabelle Arnulf, and Marie-Christine Mouren. "Iron Deficiency in Children with Attention-Deficit/Hyperactivity Disorder." *Archives of Pediatrics & Adolescent Medicine* 158, no. 12 (2004): 1113. https://doi.org/10.1001/ archpedi.158.12.1113.

Lee, Sung Kyun, Yoo Jung Park, Min Jung Ko, Ziyu Wang, Ha Young Lee, Young Whan Choi, and Yoe-Sik Bae. "A Novel Natural Compound from Garlic (Allium Sativum L.) with Therapeutic Effects Against Experimental Polymicrobial Sepsis." *Biochemical and Biophysical Research Communications* 464, no. 3 (2015): 774–9. https://doi. org/10.1016/j.bbrc.2015.07.031.

Levy, Susan E., and Susan L. Hyman. "Complementary and Alternative Medicine Treatments for Children with Autism Spectrum Disorders." *Child and Adolescent Psychiatric Clinics of North America* 24, no. 1 (2015): 117–43. https://doi. org/10.1016/j.chc.2014.09.004.

Lissiman, Elizabeth, Alice L. Bhasale, and Marc Cohen. "Garlic for the Common Cold." *Cochrane Database of Systematic Reviews*, no. 11 (2014). https://doi. org/10.1002/14651858.cd006206.pub4.

Marik, Paul E., and Joseph Varon. "Omega-3 Dietary Supplements and the Risk of Cardiovascular Events: A Systematic Review." *Clinical Cardiology* 32, no. 7 (2009): 365–72. https://doi.org/10.1002/clc.20604.

Mehrabi, Tayebe, Somayeh Gorji, Behzad Zolfaghari, and Rasool Razmjoo. "The Effect of Rosmarinus Herbal Tea on Occupational Burnout in Iran Chemical Industry Investment Company Employees." *Iranian Journal of Nursing and Midwifery Research* 20, no. 4 (2015): 460–4. https://doi.org/10.4103/1735-9066.161004.

Morey, Jennifer N., Ian A. Boggero, April B. Scott, and Suzanne C. Segerstrom. "Current Directions in Stress and Human Immune Function." *Current Opinion in Psychology* 5, (2015): 13–7. https://doi.org/10.1016/j.copsyc.2015.03.007.

Nantz, Meri P., Cheryl A. Rowe, Catherine Muller, Rebecca Creasy, Joy M. Stanilka, and Susan S. Percival. "Supplementation with Aged Garlic Extract Improves Both NK and T Cell Function and Reduces the Severity of Cold and Flu Symptoms: A Randomized, Double-blind, Placebo-controlled Nutrition Intervention." *Clinical Nutrition* 31, no. 3 (2012): 337–44. https://doi.org/10.1016/j.clnu.2011.11.019.

Rash, Joshua A., Kyle Matsuba, and Kenneth M. Prkachin. "Gratitude and Well-Being: Who Benefits the Most from a Gratitude Intervention?" *Applied Psychology: Health and Well-Being* 3, no. 3 (2011): 350–69. https://doi.org/10.1111/j.1758-0854.2011.01058.x.

Ren, Wenkai, Yinghui Li, Xinglong Yu, Wei Luo, Gang Liu, Hua Shao, and Yulong Yin. "Glutamine Modifies Immune Responses of Mice Infected with Porcine Circovirus Type 2." *British Journal of Nutrition* 110, no. 6 (2013): 1053–60. https://doi.org/10.1017/s0007114512006101.

Rennard, B. O., R. F. Ertl, G. L. Gossman, R. A. Robbins, and S. I. Rennard. "Chicken Soup Inhibits Neutrophil Chemotaxis In Vitro." *Chest* 118, no. 4 (2000): 1150–7. https://doi.org/10.1378/chest.118.4.1150.

Rucklidge, Julia J., Chris M. Frampton, Brigette Gorman, and Anna Boggis. "Vitamin–Mineral Treatment of Attention-Deficit Hyperactivity Disorder in Adults: Double-blind Randomised Placebo-controlled Trial." *British Journal of Psychiatry* 204, no. 4 (2014): 306–15. https://doi.org/10.1192/bjp.bp.113.132126.

Saxena, R. C., R. Singh, P. Kumar, S. C. Yadav, M. P. S. Negi, V. S. Saxena, A. J. Joshua, V. Vijayabalaji, K. S. Goudar, K. Venkateshwarlu, and A. Amit. "A Randomized Double Blind Placebo Controlled Clinical Evaluation of Extract of Andrographis Paniculata (Kalmcold) in Patients with Uncomplicated Upper Respiratory Tract Infection." *Phytomedicine* 17, no. 3–4 (2010): 178–85. https://doi.org/10.1016/j.phymed.2009.12.001.

Shah, Sachin A., Stephen Sander, C. Michael White, Mike Rinaldi, and Craig I. Coleman. "Evaluation of Echinacea for the Prevention and Treatment of the Common Cold: A Meta-Analysis." *The Lancet Infectious Diseases* 7, no. 7 (2007): 473–80. https://doi.org/10.1016/s1473-3099(07)70160-3.

Song, K., and J. A. Milner. "The Influence of Heating on the Anticancer Properties of Garlic." *The Journal of Nutrition* 131, no. 3 (2001): 1054S–7S. https://doi.org/10.1093/jn/131.3.1054s.

Swanson, J. M., and M. Kinsbourne. "Food Dyes Impair Performance of Hyperactive Children on a Laboratory Learning Test." *Science* 207, no. 4438 (1980): 1485–7. https://doi.org/10.1126/science.7361102.

Townsend, Elizabeth A., Matthew E. Siviski, Yi Zhang, Carrie Xu, Bhupinder Hoonjan, and Charles W. Emala. "Effects of Ginger and Its Constituents on Airway Smooth Muscle Relaxation and Calcium Regulation." *American Journal of Respiratory Cell and Molecular Biology* 48, no. 2 (2013): 157–63. https://doi.org/10.1165/rcmb.2012-0231oc.

Vasconcelos, N. G., J. Croda, and S. Simionatto. "Antibacterial Mechanisms of Cinnamon and Its Constituents: A Review." *Microbial Pathogenesis* 120, (2018): 198–203. https://doi.org/10.1016/j.micpath.2018.04.036.

Yang, Jyh-Ferng, Cheng-Hong Yang, Hsueh-Wei Chang, Cheng-San Yang, Shao-Ming Wang, Ming-Che Hsieh, and Li-Yeh Chuang. "Chemical Composition and Antibacterial Activities of Illicium Verum Against Antibiotic-resistant Pathogens." *Journal of Medicinal Food* 13, no. 5 (2010): 1254–62. https://doi.org/10.1089/jmf.2010.1086.

CPSIA information can be obtained
at www.ICGtesting.com
Printed in the USA
BVHW041318280822
645477BV00007B/95/J